CONQUER DEPRESSION

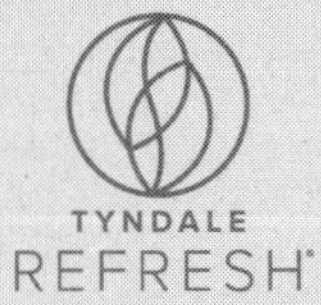

Think Well. Live Well. Be Well.

GREGORY L. JANTZ, PHD

with KEITH WALL

CONQUER DEPRESSION

7 SECRETS TO TAKE BACK YOUR LIFE

Visit Tyndale online at tyndale.com.

Tyndale and Tyndale's quill logo are registered trademarks of Tyndale House Ministries. *Tyndale Refresh* and the Tyndale Refresh logo are trademarks of Tyndale House Ministries. Tyndale Refresh is a nonfiction imprint of Tyndale House Publishers, Carol Stream, Illinois.

Conquer Depression: 7 Secrets to Take Back Your Life

Adapted from *Healing Depression for Life*, published in 2019 under ISBN 978-1-4964-3461-6.

Designed by Lindsey Bergsma

Edited by Jonathan Schindler

Published in association with The Bindery Agency, www.TheBinderyAgency.com.

For information about special discounts for bulk purchases, please contact Tyndale House Publishers at csresponse@tyndale.com, or call 1-855-277-9400.

Library of Congress Cataloging-in-Publication Data

A catalog record for this book is available from the Library of Congress.

ISBN 979-8-4005-0529-4

Printed in the United States of America

31 30 29 28 27 26 25
7 6 5 4 3 2 1

Contents

INTRODUCTION

FIND A NEW PATH FORWARD

We've all heard it before: "Depression is all in your head! Just give it time." Or worse, "Snap out of it already!"

This kind of advice is rarely loving or helpful—though, like the broken clock that is accurate twice a day, it occasionally manages to be sort of right. That is, for people who are experiencing an ordinary case of the blues or temporary emotional upheaval due to grief or trauma, time can be an ally, and natural mental resiliency usually does return in due course.

But for millions of people around the world, those more common scenarios are unfamiliar. These individuals are caught in the grip of something larger and more tenacious than that. They suffer from clinical depression, and no amount of glib advice is going to make it "go away." So here, at the beginning of our journey of conquering depression, let's orient ourselves on the map and all agree on a common starting point:

Depression is real. And painful. And frightening.

All too often, depression can even be life threatening when it drains a person of hope to the point of considering self-harm. Beyond the toll it takes on individual lives, depression places enormous strain on families, businesses, schools, and governments. In the United States, the 2016 National Survey on Drug Use and Health revealed that 16.2 million adults and 3.1 million adolescents between ages 12 and 17 had endured a recent "major depressive episode." Around two-thirds of those people suffered life impairments that were rated as "severe." However, approximately 37 percent of these adults and a staggering 60 percent of young people received no treatment of any kind, according to the survey.[1]

To make matters worse, research in recent years has revealed that, of those who do seek help, approximately one-third receive little or no lasting benefit from treatments commonly used today.[2] Think about that for a moment: one in three people sees little or no long-term benefit from common treatments for depression. Clearly, the typical approaches offer very limited lasting benefits.

According to the National Institute for Mental Health, symptoms of depression include the following:

- persistent sad, anxious, or "empty" mood
- feelings of hopelessness or pessimism

- feelings of guilt, worthlessness, or helplessness
- loss of interest or pleasure in hobbies or activities
- decreased energy, fatigue, or being "slowed down"
- difficulty concentrating, remembering, or making decisions
- difficulty sleeping, early-morning awakening, or oversleeping
- appetite and/or weight changes
- thoughts of death or suicide or suicide attempts
- restlessness or irritability
- persistent physical symptoms such as aches or indigestion[3]

At The Center: A Place of Hope, the clinic where I work, we believe that if a person reports a chronic combination of these symptoms lasting sixty to ninety days—far beyond what's expected in cases of the ordinary blues we all experience from time to time—then they are in need of coordinated care for major depression. Our admissions specialists assess the severity of depression in those seeking help using three criteria: hopelessness, helplessness, and despair. Once a person's experience can be characterized by words as bleak as these, they have long lost the ability to "snap out of it."

That so many people do reach this point in their lives makes depression a human tragedy of stunning proportions.

Treatment Is a Team Effort

Now that we've established the magnitude of the problem, let's agree on a vastly more important fact: *it doesn't have to be this way.* Healing is possible, now and for good.

If that's the case, why do our treatment methods continue to fall so short? Why do even the lucky ones with access to care so often come away disappointed?

While the answers to these questions are far from simple, they also don't take an advanced degree in medicine to understand. There is a certain lack of common sense at the root of the problem. Care providers tend to use their favorite depression treatments as singular fixes for a disorder that is never caused by one thing alone. In my experience, depression always arises from multiple factors converging in a person's life. Treating one thing at a time, with one method at a time, is akin to expecting new tires to revitalize a car with multiple systems on the blink.

More than thirty years of practice and experience at The Center: A Place of Hope have led us to some compelling conclusions about why most isolated depression treatments are failing. The nation is losing ground in its battle with depression, due in part to one or more of the following:

Over-prescription and misuse of medication. In The Center's early years, we saw clients who had tried or were currently taking no more than two or three medications. These days, our average incoming client is taking five different medications or more. Often these drugs contribute to the problem or create new issues. More troubling, these multiple medications sometimes compete dangerously with each other in the patient's body or combine in unpredictable ways. And that's before accounting for side effects the pharmaceutical companies have already identified.

In fact, a recent study found that one-third of adults in the US may be unknowingly using prescription drugs that could cause depression or increase the risk of suicide. As one report stated, "Over 200 commonly prescribed drugs carry warnings that depression or suicide are potential side effects. But patients and clinicians may be unaware of this link because the drugs may treat conditions unrelated to depression or mental health."[4] Indeed, many medications can lead to serious physical symptoms, which are often treated with—you guessed it—more medication!

Relying completely on medication as the solution. When general practitioners prescribe psychotropic medications without the input of a psychiatrist or other mental health specialist, and when patients request medications based on self-diagnosis drawn from internet research or a TV-commercial-fueled desire for a certain brand of medication, we often see a person given an antidepressant when they're really suffering from an anxiety disorder (and vice versa). Medication is too often perceived as a quick fix, to the exclusion of other possible—and necessary—care.

One-dimensional treatment answers. There's an old saying: "If all you have is a hammer, everything looks like a nail." In the context of medical care, that means physicians who are trained to think that all disease is the result of a biochemical malfunction in the body will naturally reach for one-time "magic pill" fixes, excluding other options. I should say that I have high regard for skilled, compassionate physicians. But my work with hundreds of depressed clients has caused me great concern about the typical medical model of treatment. Often medical practitioners ignore alternative causes for chronic depression and quickly prescribe a pill as the cure-all. Despite current research showing that many other wellness factors affect our mood—such as gut health, sleep patterns, and behavioral habits—a disappointing majority of professionals continue to limit analysis and treatment to what's going on in a patient's gray matter.

Toxic emotions. Before reaching for typical medical treatments, it's important to examine what I call the "three deadly emotions"—anger, fear, and guilt. Chances are if someone is struggling with depression, they are also suffering from the unhealthy influence of one or more of these emotions, which fuel depressive tendencies and can hinder treatment by other methods.

One of the most universal contributing factors to depression in our clients—which is often not explored by other treatment providers—is entrenched resentment or an inability to forgive. The negative emotions that linger when a person hasn't forgiven someone can create a state of chronic depression, which damages the body on multiple levels. We have seen such strong evidence that these factors play key roles in depression that our treatment approach routinely includes shining a light on those dark, secret places.

Distractions and addictions. While technology has enabled us to create more community ties and stay in touch with far-flung loved ones, the disturbing and largely unexplored reality is that technology also promotes distinct patterns of isolation and social conflict that contribute to depression. Many of our guests at The Center exhibit all the signs of withdrawal from a physical addiction after just a few days without their electronic devices.

Diet. Few people are aware that common chemicals in our diet, like artificial sweeteners and preservatives, are actually neurotoxins that build up in the body and interfere with our health. In treating depression, it's vital to examine what we are putting into our bodies to ensure that it is helping our efforts to heal rather than hindering them.

A Way Out of the Dark

When searching for effective ways to treat and heal from depression, we should be looking not for the one smoking gun but rather for all the missing puzzle pieces. Conquering depression can only be achieved through integrated, multifaceted approaches that give attention to the whole person.

In the coming chapters, we will look at the whole person to discover what factors might be contributing to your depression and how you can holistically address them. Each chapter is oriented around practical changes that, when implemented together, will help you heal. While it may be tempting to jump around, and while the chapters can be read independently, I would encourage you to view them as a whole treatment plan. As already discussed, treatment is a team effort, and just as it is helpful when looking at individual puzzle pieces to see the picture on the box, you will likely have a better understanding of yourself and your needs if you are armed with all the information in this book.

If you are suffering from depression, or someone you love is, chances are you've come to this book because you've tried other options that left you disappointed and discouraged. The purpose of this chapter is to say, "Take heart!" If previous treatments have not worked for you, the fault does not lie with you but with the common—and mistaken—belief that any *one* drug or process can hold all the answers. As you now know, the most effective treatment attacks depression on multiple fronts. Take heart, because the rest of this book will show you how to succeed in conquering depression where other attempts have let you down.

1

EAT AND DRINK WHAT IS GOOD

Every gardener knows that plants can't grow without the essential elements of water, light, and properly balanced soil. If you have too much water, you will drown your plants. Too little, and they will starve. Too little light, and they will wither. Too much, and they will burn. As for the soil, only the appropriate balance of nutrients and minerals will allow your garden to thrive.

Our bodies respond in the same way. Without the proper balance of the right elements, our bodies will not thrive. And when

I say "our bodies," this of course means *everything* about our physical makeup: our brain function, metabolism, muscle tone, bone strength, energy level, immune system efficiency, sexual vitality, digestive health, and on and on. And when I say "the right elements," this means proper nutrition and hydration—food and drink that empowers the body to function at its optimal capacity. The right food will provide the right results.

We sometimes hear it said of Olympic athletes or others who physically perform at a high level, "Her body is a well-oiled machine!" I have news for you: God created *your* body to be a well-oiled machine, too, whether or not you run marathons, swim a hundred laps every day, or cycle long distances. The psalmist had a more poetic description of the human body, saying we are "fearfully and wonderfully made" by our Creator (Psalm 139:14). Your body and mind form an intricate, delicate system . . . and this system is fueled and fortified by nutrient-rich foods also wonderfully made by our Creator. God designed our bodies and the earth's rich food sources to work in harmony, bringing us maximum health and wellness.

Here's the key point: nutritious, fortifying foods support not only physical health but mental health as well. What you put in your mouth each day affects your mood and mental health directly and dramatically.

The Gut and the Brain

An emerging body of research has linked mental health with the gut. To make it really simple: the vagus nerve is our body's biggest nerve, running from the brain down to the gut, where it branches into a vast information network of neurons. This two-lane highway, along with our immune system and hormones, is known as the gut-brain axis. In the past, it was thought that this system's purpose was for the brain to more closely monitor and control digestive functions, which are among the most complex operations in the body.

But some studies have revealed that 90 percent of the fibers in the vagus nerve are actually sending messages *from* this intricate system of neurons *to the brain*, and not the other way around. Even more interesting is that this system uses more than thirty neurotransmitters, as many as the "big" brain uses, to send these signals, underscoring the relationship between the gut and mood disorders, which are typically related to the body's ability to produce, absorb, and use certain neurotransmitters such as serotonin.

Let me put it plainly: your gut sends messages to your brain that directly influence your level of anxiety, happiness, satisfaction, and depression.

For the first time in modern history, a wealth of medical research is supporting a view that the brain is not, in fact, the root of all mood disorders, and that opens up whole new avenues for treating depression and related disorders.[1]

Proper nutrition is, therefore, an essential aspect of managing depression. Some foods are extremely beneficial to our overall health as well as our mental health. Likewise, some foods are detrimental, negatively affecting our moods. It's important to understand that being careful about what you put into your body can go a long way toward conquering your depression.

Foods That Contribute to Depression

While much could be said about the benefits and tools of good nutrition, I want to highlight some basic yet essential guidelines related to nutrition and depression. We will focus on what foods actually *contribute to* depression and what foods help *combat* its debilitating effects. That is the good news: there are foods and liquids that have been scientifically proven to help fend off depression.

Let's start with what we *don't* want to put in our bodies. Below are some of the main culprits leading to nutritional imbalance. A phrase I often use to point out the five main mischief-makers in our culture's diet is "devitalized food." The "Big 5" include:

1. Processed foods
2. Junk foods
3. White flour
4. White rice
5. Refined sugar

You'll notice that most of the elements I mention above are white in color—all processed and all bad for you. And devitalized foods are often the most tempting: the quick burger and fries at the drive-thru as you rush home exhausted after a long day. Or those cookies on the grocery store shelf that taste so good as you relax in front of the TV at night.

They are hard to resist. But if we are serious about conquering depression, we need to wage war on the worst dietary offenders. Yes, it may mean cooking after a long day when you don't feel like it. Or it may mean eating foods that don't have the same sweet-and-savory "zing" as those deep-fried foods that deliver empty calories and bad ingredients.

The devitalized foods and drinks I refer to provide only *fragmented* nutrition, meaning they contain only a small amount of what your body needs. Right alongside fragmented foods (such as the "white foods" mentioned above) are their equally destructive cousins, the junk foods. Common ingredients in junk foods include additives, preservatives, pumped-up or masked sugars, fats, salts, artificial colors, and food dyes.

Like many things when it comes to human biology and physiology, everyone is different. While some people can drink a cup of coffee at 11:00 p.m. and fall right to sleep, others stay awake all night if they've had caffeine eight hours before bedtime. But there are general rules to follow and foods and beverages to avoid if you are struggling with depression. Here are the main types:

1. **Caffeine.** Not only can caffeine be addictive, but once the thrill is gone, it might even exacerbate your depression by making you more anxious and nervous.
2. **Alcohol.** This is a depressant, which means it reduces your brain's serotonin, a neurotransmitter that acts as a mood stabilizer. Alcohol can also act as a stimulant and increase anxiety and stress.
3. **Additives.** I want to highlight two particularly unhealthy additives that are in a surprising number of

foods and beverages: monosodium glutamate (MSG) and aspartame. Studies have shown that aspartame—a common artificial sweetener—can cause DNA damage, increase obesity, and contribute to depression symptoms. MSG, like aspartame, may also interfere with the balance of neurotransmitters in your brain, leading to depression.

4. **Processed foods.** Stay away from processed foods as much as possible, including hot dogs, most deli meats (unless organic and fresh), and fried foods. Another subtle culprit: margarine. Stick to real butter, as margarine is high in unhealthy trans-fatty acids, along with coloring additives and emulsifiers.
5. **Refined sugars.** Avoid foods high in refined sugar, like cookies, most juices, and of course candy. The

trouble is they have a detrimental effect on your blood sugar levels as they contain no fiber. This means that when your system is flush with refined sugar, it causes your glucose levels to fluctuate dramatically, which in turn can lead to anxiousness, irritability, and depression.

Foods That Help Relieve Depression

It would be nice if medical science identified a quick-fix "magic formula" for combating depression through nutrition. Unfortunately, nutritional eating isn't quite that simple . . . but neither is it overly complex. It often comes down to common sense. You know a party-size bag of potato chips and a liter of cherry soda will taste great while you watch the football game, but you also know this taste-bud-tantalizing snack will deliver only empty calories.

Maybe you should listen to the wise words your mother used to tell you when you were growing up: "Eat your fruits and vegetables . . . and stay away from cake and candy." By steering you toward plants and away from sweets, Mom was definitely pointing you in the right direction.

Let's consider a nutrition-rich diet that will help relieve your depression. Everyone likes the idea of "eating healthy," but what does that look like day in and day out? Here are several helpful strategies—along with specific food recommendations—that will enrich your body and lift your mood.[2]

Be "carb conscious." Serotonin, the mood-altering brain chemical, has been shown to be affected by carbohydrates. Researchers speculate that an individual's craving for carbs is related to low serotonin activity. What's more, some carbs have been shown to have a calming effect, while others do not. It's best to avoid sugary foods and to consume "smart" or "complex" carbs (such as whole grains) rather than simple carbs, often found in baked goods.

Provide your brain with healthy proteins. The amino acid tryptophan (found in turkey, tuna, chicken, and similar foods) boosts your brain's production of serotonin. So try to eat protein-rich foods several times a day, especially when your energy level needs a lift. Healthy choices include beans and peas, lean beef, low-fat cheese, fish, milk, poultry, soy products, and yogurt. As I've said elsewhere, avoid processed proteins—such as packaged lunch meats and wrapped cheese slices—and look for organic choices instead.

Be "vitamin B aware." Several research studies have demonstrated the link between vitamin B_{12} deficiency and depression. B vitamins can be found in legumes, nuts, many fruits, dark green vegetables, and low-fat animal products, such as fish and low-fat dairy products.

Make vitamin D a must-have. In a 2013 meta-analysis, researchers concluded that a deficiency in vitamin D results in a higher risk of suffering from depression. Because vitamin D is essential to the brain, low levels of it can be a factor in depression and other mental illnesses. To ensure you're getting enough vitamin D, consume plenty of salmon, egg yolks, yogurt, whole milk, almond milk, orange juice, oatmeal, cheese, shiitake mushrooms, and fortified tofu.

Optimize your diet with omega-3 fatty acids. According to researchers, major depressive disorders occur at higher rates among those who are lacking in omega-3s, and depression is more likely to occur in people who seldom eat fish (a common source of omega-3s). Good sources of omega-3s include fatty fish (anchovy, mackerel, salmon, sardines, shad, and tuna), flaxseed, canola and soybean oils, nuts (especially walnuts), and dark green leafy vegetables.

Find more fiber. Replace foods high in sugar and fat with those high in fiber. This includes vegetables such as asparagus, Jerusalem artichokes, broccoli, Brussels sprouts, cabbage, cauliflower, collard greens, kale, leeks, and onions, as well as bananas, legumes, and nuts. This also includes whole grains, such as barley, whole wheat, and oats. Fiber plays an important role in regulating your digestive system and helping you feel fuller so you have fewer cravings.

Replace Unhealthy with Healthy Drinks

We've looked at some general guidelines for nutritional eating. What about drinks? Here are some ideas of healthy swaps you can make.

Instead of caffeine-based coffee and black tea, *swap with* herbal and green teas with less or no caffeine, or decaf coffee, black. Also try chamomile, lemon balm, peppermint, rosemary, and turmeric tea, the latter of which has been used for centuries in Chinese medicine as a treatment for depression.

Instead of a steady intake of alcoholic drinks high in sugars, such as spirits, *swap with* red wine, particularly drier reds, which are lower in sugar content than sweeter wines, such as white chardonnays. If you are going to drink hard alcohol, such as vodka, gin, tequila, or whiskey, avoid or limit mixed drinks that add sugar, such as daiquiris, piña coladas, margaritas, and so on. (I mention this substitution because I know some people will consume alcohol even if I, and others, advise against it for those struggling with depression.)

Instead of sodas and sugary "fruit juices," *swap with* organic juices containing 100 percent real juice. Or try kombucha, a drink that is made through the fermentation of sweet tea with a culture of yeast and good bacteria.

And as we think about healthy drinks, let's not overlook one of the most essential components of nutrition: water. Ever since you were in grade school, you've heard that H_2O is an indispensable element of the earth's ecosystem, necessary for sustaining every aspect of life—plants, trees, animals, oceans, weather systems, and human beings. Water, of course, is also an indispensable element for our individual bodies if we hope to survive and thrive.

In the United States, there is little risk that you will not *survive* because of lack of water . . . but it's that second word we can focus on: *thrive*.

Scientists have identified a strong connection between dehydration and depression, noting that even mild dehydration will affect your moods. Proper water intake also helps to support weight loss, maintain muscle mass, sustain kidney function, and aid digestion.[3]

So how much water consumption will help you thrive? You've probably heard that you should drink at least eight eight-ounce glasses of water each day (i.e., sixty-four ounces). Well, there is a lot of truth to that. Don't forget that our bodies are composed of approximately 60 percent water. We need a lot of water to keep our biological machine humming along in good health.

Actually, what I advise my clients is that they drink the equivalent of half their body weight in ounces of water each day. For example, if you weigh 176 pounds, you should drink 88 ounces per day—the equivalent of eleven eight-ounce glasses of water. The trick is to start early in the morning and have a water container near you during the day—even while you are driving.

And just to be clear: I am talking about *water*, not just *liquids*. So if you have juice or coffee with lunch, don't count those ounces toward your daily water intake. Remember that a lot of the liquids we rely on each day—coffee, soda, black tea, beer—contain either caffeine or alcohol, both of which are diuretics. In other words, they actually do the *opposite* of what water does: they dehydrate you rather than hydrate you.

—

Any strategy for conquering depression should include examining what you eat and drink. You've probably heard the saying that "you are what you eat," and with nutritious food and drinks that combat depression (rather than exacerbating it), you will be one step closer to your goal.

2

GET MOVING

If Gina didn't set an alarm for 2:40 in the afternoon, the chances were good that she would forget to pick up her daughter from kindergarten.

Gina was deeply depressed, and her emotions and behaviors showed it. She felt sad and numb. She had little energy for the tasks of daily life. Most days, she woke up long enough to drive her daughter, Lexie, to school; then she came home and slept or stared out the picture window in the living room until it was time to pick Lexie up. As soon as dinner was over, Gina would crawl back under the covers, leaving her husband, Steve, to finish out the evening with their five-year-old.

One day Steve begged Gina to take an online depression screening, and neither was surprised when her scores indicated she was clinically depressed.

The couple came to The Center: A Place of Hope convinced that Gina needed to start on antidepressants. After visiting with the two of them and reviewing medical history and lab work, Gina's physician said, "You could go on antidepressants, but I believe walking for thirty minutes five times a week will do as much good or more as medication."

A lot was going on in Gina's life, body, and brain that had been contributing to her depression, and the whole-person plan we designed for her tackled the problem from many angles. But a critical part of that plan was getting Gina moving again.

The idea that exercise can alleviate and even prevent depression is not new. Neither is the idea that, in some cases, exercise can be as effective as antidepressants in stabilizing or improving moods.

In one study, 156 adults with major depressive disorder were randomized into three groups. The first group participated in aerobic exercise sessions three times a week; the second group was given an antidepressant; and the third group participated in a combination of exercise and medication.

After four months, the group that participated in exercise alone benefited *as much as the other two groups.* It's especially interesting that participants in the exercise-only group were also less likely to relapse into depression, and those who exercised regularly during a ten-month follow-up period were less likely (by more than 50 percent) than non-exercisers to be depressed.[1]

The study is one of many with similar

findings. In fact, professors from the University of Toronto analyzed twenty-six years of research on the link between depression and exercise. Their conclusion was that even low levels of physical activity for twenty to thirty minutes a day could reduce or prevent depression in people of all ages.[2]

Start Somewhere

I have to admit that when I'm talking with our clients, I often substitute a different term for the word *exercise*. Some people associate the word with such grueling discomfort or past monumental efforts and failures that they immediately resist the idea.

Instead, I use the phrase "physical movement."

Instead of telling depressed clients to begin an exercise program, I talk to them about moving more and increasing their activity. Many depressed individuals have such low energy and low motivation that exercise is the last thing they want to do.

One of my clients found exercising such a daunting challenge that she discovered a *very* gradual way to get started. She simply made it her daily goal to get dressed in her gym clothes, drive to the gym, and stand on the treadmill. That was all.

Well, it was a start. If she did those three things, she considered her goals met for the day. This effectively eliminated the "I'm too tired" excuse. Whenever she had that thought, she reminded herself that she didn't have to actually *do* anything; she just had to stand on the treadmill, which of course took little effort.

Her strategy also took care of the "I don't have time to work out" excuse. Whenever she had that thought, she reminded herself she didn't have to spend much time at the gym—she just had to stand for a moment on the treadmill, which of course took little time at all.

You can imagine what happened next. More often than not, by the time this woman drove to the gym and stood on the treadmill, her next thought was, *As long as I'm here, I might as well walk for ten minutes.* In the weeks ahead, ten minutes became twenty, then forty, and by the end of the year she had lost twenty pounds, had improved her eating habits, and was sleeping better at night. Her energy level had rebounded, along with her self-esteem. Her symptoms of depression did not magically vanish altogether, but she felt the renewed vitality and optimism to begin addressing other aspects of her life that would lead her toward healing.

This woman was wise in discerning that she needed to train her schedule and her willpower before she began training her body. And it worked. By starting slow, we give our bodies, routines, and self-discipline time to catch up to what our brains know we need to do. The important thing is to begin doing *something*, no matter how small or simple.

The Magic Hour

To combat depression, you don't need to hire a personal trainer or spend hours at the gym (although I would encourage both options). You can improve your mobility and mental health by consistently choosing to move more in simple ways. For example, try parking a little farther from your workplace, taking the stairs instead of the elevator, walking the dog after dinner, spending thirty minutes a day gardening, or meeting a friend several times a week for a stroll through a park.

A study published in the *American Journal of Psychiatry* followed 33,908 healthy adults for eleven years and tracked data related to exercise, depression, and anxiety. The researchers concluded that sedentary participants were

44 percent more likely to develop depression than participants who exercised just one to two hours a week. In fact, that one-hour mark was particularly significant. Here are some of the conclusions of the study:

- When it came to protecting people from depression, most of the benefits were realized with an hour of low-level exercise a week.
- Low-intensity exercises were just as beneficial as high-intensity exercises.
- Future cases of depression could have been prevented among 12 percent of the study's participants if they had engaged in at least one hour of physical activity each week.[3]

The benefits of even moderate physical activity are widespread and substantial. According to Dr. Alpa Patel, strategic director of the American Cancer Society's Cancer Prevention Study-3, "When you go from doing no activity to any amount, you see a marked decline in the risk of premature death from any cause."[4] I am struck by that amazing sequence of words: *any amount . . . marked decline . . . from any cause.*

Of course, there are additional benefits from consistent workouts of higher intensity. According to the Physical Activity Guidelines for Americans, your weekly activity goal should include two and a half hours of moderate-intensity aerobic activity (such as brisk walking) and two days of muscle-strengthening activities that work all major muscle groups (legs, hips, back, abs, chest, shoulders, and arms). Meeting these guidelines can literally save your life, creating dramatic improvements related to diabetes, heart health, bone and muscle strength, and more.[5]

But studies show that when it comes to mental health, increasing your activity level even a small amount—especially if you've been sedentary—matters. A lot.

The "Magic Pill"

Clients of mine who start moving—and then stay moving as a cornerstone of a healthier lifestyle—are more successful at reducing or eliminating symptoms of depression, now and in the future. And yet the benefits of moving more don't stop there.

"Exercise is the magic pill," says Dr. Michael Bracko, chairman of the American College of Sports Medicine's Consumer Information Committee, adding that "exercise can literally cure diseases like some forms of heart disease. Exercise has been implicated in helping people prevent or recover from some forms of cancer. Exercise helps people with arthritis. Exercise helps people prevent and reverse depression."[6]

You already know that exercise is good

for your whole body, including your mental health. But let me highlight some specific health benefits here. Physical movement helps to . . .

- **Strengthen bones.** Weight-bearing exercises strengthen muscles by causing new bone tissue to grow. When you think of weight-bearing exercises, you may think immediately of lifting weights, but "weight-bearing exercises" also refers to movements that cause you to support the weight of your own body. These include walking, jogging, climbing stairs, dancing, and even jumping.
- **Build muscles.** Muscle-building exercises are increasingly important as we age, as the human body begins losing muscle mass from about the age of thirty. When we refuse to let nature take its course and become

intentional about moving in ways that help us maintain and even build muscle, we reap the benefits in nearly every area of life. Besides the obvious perks, stronger muscles improve balance and reduce the likelihood of falls as we age and help maintain bone mass, reducing our chances of developing osteoporosis.

- **Provide a better night's sleep.** We will examine the link between depression and sleep in the next chapter, but getting a solid night's sleep can dramatically improve emotional health. According to one study, people with chronic insomnia who engaged in medium-intensity aerobic exercise (such as walking) fell asleep quicker and slept longer.[7]
- **Support cardiovascular health.** Every year, about 735,000 American adults have a heart attack. In fact, heart

disease is the leading cause of death for men and women, killing more than 600,000 people in the United States every year.[8] Study after study shows that physical inactivity is a significant risk factor for heart disease and that exercise can dramatically reduce your risk of developing heart disease—and can even help reverse damage that has already occurred. Four of the best exercises for a healthy heart are brisk walking, running, swimming, and bicycling.

- **Lower blood sugar.** Exercise lowers blood sugar by increasing insulin sensitivity. This helps your muscle cells use available insulin to take up glucose during and after your workout. The contraction of your muscles during exercise also improves the way your cells absorb and use glucose, even without insulin.[9]

In addition to doing wonders for your brain and body, physical movement can be a game changer when it comes to your overall attitude and mind-set. Dr. John Ratey, author of the book *Spark: The Revolutionary New Science of Exercise and the Brain*, says exercise is the perfect tool for reprogramming a depressed prefrontal cortex. It can reprogram how you think and cope too. Here's what else regular movement is going to do for you:

- **Increase your confidence.** There's the confidence that comes from having a body that is fit and healthy, and there is also confidence that comes from doing something every day that you know is good for you. Either way, regular physical movement empowers you to feel better about yourself.
- **Boost your creativity.** Research conducted at Stanford University

showed that something as simple as casual walking improves creativity by boosting convergent thinking (solving a problem) as well as divergent thinking (coming up with original ideas).[10]

- **Help you cope.** The endorphins released while exercising serve as your body's natural painkillers while helping to reduce anxiety and stress. That makes exercise the perfect go-to activity when you're looking for a healthy coping strategy.

Ready, Set, Go!

When I told Gina to begin her journey to wellness by placing one foot in front of the other, she resisted. Tearing up, she told me she had neither the energy nor the desire to move more than she already did . . . which amounted to getting herself to the car and back a couple of times a day.

But a few weeks later, when a neighbor suggested a short walk every morning after Gina returned from taking Lexie to school, Gina agreed to get outside her comfort zone and muster the energy to start slowly.

The first three mornings, the two women walked just a few blocks. Gina had been afraid that her neighbor would be frustrated by the slow pace and short distance. But she soon discovered that her neighbor had her own struggles and was filled with nothing but compassion and understanding for Gina.

Gina opted for consistency over intensity. She focused more on getting out her front door every morning rather than pushing herself to walk farther than she felt comfortable. Within a week, the two women were walking twice as far—plus, Gina realized their growing companionship and daily conversation provided much-needed support as she began to slowly navigate her way out of the darkness and into the light. In the months ahead, this consistent physical movement, and the camaraderie that came with it, became a cornerstone of Gina's healing.

Exercise is such a powerful resource because the impact is so comprehensive. In fact, time after time, I see the power of movement become a catalyst for transformation in many areas in my clients' lives.

So, when you're finished with this chapter, take a break from your reading and go for a walk or a bike ride. Start moving, and soon you'll find your emotional health improving.

3

DEVELOP A SLEEP ROUTINE

Jennifer used to love her life. She had a challenging career as a software developer, a husband and three children she adored, and a supportive network of family and friends. Her family lived in a nice home in a Dallas suburb with frequent block parties and barbecues. Jennifer's life seemed picture perfect, and for a long time she would have agreed with that description.

Then everything changed.

Looking back, she could pinpoint when the shift occurred. She remembered a five-month period during which grief was her constant companion. Losing a childhood friend to breast cancer and a colleague to suicide five weeks later left Jennifer reeling. A few months later, the death of her ninety-two-year-old grandmother, while not unexpected, was another huge loss. That fall, when Jennifer's seven-year-old son was diagnosed with type 1 diabetes, something in Jennifer felt broken beyond repair.

And so began a two-year spiral that culminated in Jennifer coming to The Center desperate for relief. In my first consultation with Jennifer, I asked her to describe her symptoms. In addition to fatigue, alternative bouts of feeling sad and numb, and being unable to focus at work, she told me she was suffering from insomnia. For several months, her sleep routine had been disrupted as she woke up nearly every night at three o'clock, only to stare at the ceiling and listen to her husband's steady breathing beside her as he slept soundly. Sometimes she would eventually fall back to sleep, sometimes not. In the morning she would get up, bleary eyed and foggy headed, and "trudge through the day like a zombie," as she described it.

Each night, Jennifer would face the same miserable scenario all over again, like a dreadful recurring scene from the movie *Groundhog Day*. Naturally, as her sleep problems persisted week after week, her depression worsened.

Although I felt deeply sympathetic as Jennifer explained her desperate situation, I wasn't at all surprised. Over several decades of working with depressed individuals, I've come to recognize that the vast majority of them suffer from sleep issues that turn into sleep disorders. It seems like a cruel irony: at a time when these people are struggling to regain stability and find a shred of hope, peaceful and restorative sleep eludes them.

The relationship between sleep and depression isn't discussed as often as, say, symptoms of sadness or fatigue. And yet, after working with literally thousands of depressed patients, I know that sleep is virtually always a part of the problem and, more important, must be an integral part of the solution.

An Epidemic of Sleep Problems

A study by the CDC shows that more than a third of adults and more than two-thirds of teenagers do not get enough sleep.[1] Undoubtedly, you've had your own experiences with sleepless nights, so the intensity of this problem is probably not surprising to you.

What may come as a surprise, however, is the pervasiveness of the problem, as well as one of the driving forces behind it. The decline in sleep quality for Americans has been called nothing short of an epidemic, and one of the dynamics fueling this epidemic is our ever-growing obsession with technology (a topic we will discuss in chapter 5).

A 2011 poll by the National Sleep Foundation revealed some disturbing trends. The study showed that nearly four in ten Americans regularly bring their cell phones into their bedrooms and use them right before trying to fall asleep. The numbers skyrocket to roughly seven in ten when we look specifically at teens and adults under the age of thirty.[2]

Why is this bad news? Let's look at the impact of something as seemingly harmless as texting right before bedtime. According to the same National Sleep Foundation poll, people who text in the hour before trying to fall asleep even a few nights a week are

- less likely to report getting a good night's sleep,
- more likely to wake up feeling unrefreshed,
- more likely to be categorized as "sleepy" on the Epworth Sleepiness Scale, and
- more likely to drive drowsy.[3]

Another dynamic that must be considered is the rise in prescription drug use. A study by researchers at the Mayo Clinic revealed that seven out of ten Americans take a prescription drug, and one in five US patients is on five or more prescription drugs—many of which include insomnia among their side effects.[4]

The fact that some medications disrupt sleep cycles is an important piece in the puzzle. Offending drugs can include medications related to past illnesses as well as concurrent illnesses and even a morass of depression medications that may have unwanted side effects. The list of prescription medications that can interfere with a healthy night's sleep includes heart medications, asthma medications, antidepressants, and nicotine patches, as well as medications for ADHD and hypothyroidism. Over-the-counter pain medications and decongestants have also been linked with insomnia.

Why does this matter? It matters because

when we don't get enough sleep, our bodies, brains, and emotions are impacted, and we experience the following:

- decreased overall activity in the brain, affecting learning, memory, attention, and productivity
- impaired driving performance and response times like the impairments experienced while driving intoxicated
- interference with healthy heart function
- compromises in how your body repairs joint and muscle injuries
- reduced production of the hormones your body uses to control appetite, leading to increased obesity

As if these outcomes weren't disruptive enough, when we consider what research continues to reveal about the link between inadequate sleep and depression and even suicidal ideations, we can no longer underestimate the healing power of sleep in the life of anyone suffering in a depressive state.

A Downward Spiral

If you've ever struggled—or struggle now—to get a good night's sleep, you know how frustrating and discouraging it can be. And you're not alone. If you ask virtually any depressed person about sleep, you will almost certainly hear about distorted and disturbed sleep patterns:

- Among people diagnosed with depression, three out of four struggle with insomnia, while 15 percent report symptoms of hypersomnia (excessive sleepiness during the day, which can occur on its own or with insomnia).
- Nearly 90 percent of people with severe depression struggle with early-morning insomnia.

- Among people who are not depressed, the presence of insomnia indicates a higher risk for depression later in life.[5]

Why are sleep issues so prevalent among people suffering from depression? Sleep studies done with depressed patients have shown that depression changes our sleep architecture. People who are depressed experience an altered sleep cycle, entering REM sleep more quickly and spending less time in sleep stages three and four.[6] Sleep stages three and four—the stages associated with delta, or slow-wave, brain activity—are often called "priority sleep" because they are so critical to our emotional and physical well-being.

The link between sleep patterns and depression is so prevalent that at The Center our team performs a sleep study with most incoming patients to help determine just how much their sleep quality has deteriorated. But the data is a tricky business. That's because it can be difficult to determine whether a person's sleep issues are symptoms of their depression or whether trouble sleeping has contributed to the rise of depression. It's a chicken-and-egg kind of dilemma: Does a person's depression cause sleep disruption, or does lack of sleep cause depression?

The answer is yes, both. What's more, I have concluded that it doesn't matter which came first, sleep disturbances or depression. Each fuels the other, creating a vicious downward spiral. The critical issue is to improve sleep quality so that depression levels will improve as well.

Sleep Hygiene: A Natural Approach

Depression and sleep deficits are unarguably entwined. Yet in that interwoven relationship lie opportunities for treatment, relief, and healing. Indeed, when you take measures to improve the quality of a depressed person's sleep, you also relieve symptoms of their depression.

At The Center, we gravitate toward the use of natural, nondrug methods to address sleep issues in our depressed clients. While our doctors are not strictly opposed to the use of medications to promote sleep, there is always the possibility that some patients will become psychologically dependent on over-the-counter sleep aids (like Sominex or Tylenol PM). There is also an addictive quality to prescription sleep meds such as Lunesta and Ambien.

This is why I prefer recommending simple, natural methods that have proven to be effective at improving sleep. These methods make up something called *sleep hygiene*, which is the term used to describe behaviors we can adopt that help to promote good sleep.

Below I recommend eleven behaviors you can adopt that will improve the quality of your sleep. You'll notice that the actions on this list don't take place only at night. This is because a good night's sleep doesn't begin an hour or two before bed but is determined by many choices, habits, and behaviors throughout the day. There are many things you can do during your waking hours that will greatly improve the quality of your sleep.

During the Day

1. **Get exposure to natural light.** Exposure to sunlight helps maintain a healthy sleep cycle. In fact, receiving intervals of light and darkness is the method by which our bodies determine our circadian rhythm, or internal clock. Exposure to natural light during the day is especially important for people who may not venture outside much.
2. **Exercise.** Just ten minutes of daily aerobic activity can significantly

improve your sleep. Because rigorous exercise circulates endorphins into the body, which can make it harder to fall asleep, I recommend getting your exercise in before midafternoon every day.

3. **Take short naps.** While some experts advise against napping because of potential disruption of nighttime sleep patterns, I encourage my clients to catch up on their slumber any time they can. Napping may not make up for a poor night's sleep, but a short nap can still be beneficial. I recommend limiting daytime naps to a half hour, however, so sleeping at night is not compromised.
4. **Review the medications you are taking.** If you suspect that sleep issues are related to a medication you are taking, talk to your physician or pharmacist. Switching medications,

changing a dosage, or taking your medication at a different time of day may be options.

As Evening Approaches

1. **Watch what you eat close to bedtime.** It's no secret that heavy, rich, or spicy foods can keep you awake at night. Even citrus fruits and carbonated drinks can trigger indigestion, and too much alcohol close to bedtime can disrupt sleep as the body processes it. In other words, when it comes to eating and drinking before bed, go easy on anything you consume.
2. **Avoid stimulants close to bedtime.** Coffee is an obvious stimulant, but many people forget that soda and tea can contain caffeine as well. Nicotine and exercise are other

stimulants that can keep us from falling quickly into sleep.

I also put emotionally upsetting conversations and activities in this category, as well as exposure to electronics. Even something as innocuous as texting right before bed provides light and stimulation that will undermine the quality of your sleep.

3. **Follow a regular, relaxing bedtime routine.** Maintaining a consistent nightly routine helps the body recognize when it's time to sleep. Your process might include taking a warm shower or bath, reading a book, or listening to soothing music. Your routine should also include going to bed and waking up around the same time. Ideally, you should go to bed and wake up within the same thirty-minute window every day.

4. **Create a comfortable environment.** As evening approaches, make sure you have arranged a peaceful, calming sleep environment. Things that help create this atmosphere may include buying a comfortable mattress and keeping your bedroom cool (between sixty and sixty-eight degrees). It can also include things like earplugs, white noise machines, humidifiers, and fans. And if you have pets that wake you up at night, keep them out of the bedroom.
5. **Don't watch TV, study, or read in bed.** When you engage in these activities, your brain associates your bed with wakefulness. Just as regular, relaxing bedtime routines can help your brain and body know when it's time for sleep, your bed itself is another important trigger. By helping your brain associate your

bed with sleep, the transition into slumber will be much smoother.

At Night

1. **Keep your room as dark as possible.** Remember, our bodies use exposure to light and dark to set our internal clocks. Even small amounts of light from lamps, cell phones, TV screens, and digital clocks will interfere. If needed, consider purchasing blackout curtains for your bedroom.
2. **Don't stay in bed awake for more than five to ten minutes.** We all experience times when we find ourselves awake in the middle of the night. Perhaps the mind is racing or we are worried about not being able to sleep or we find ourselves wide awake for no discernible reason at all. Given the need to train our brains

> to associate our beds with sleeping, lying awake in bed for hours is rarely a good idea. Instead, if you can't fall back asleep within five or ten minutes, get out of bed and sit in a chair in the dark until you feel sleepy, and then climb back in bed. And whatever you do, don't pick up your phone or turn on the TV. The light will confuse your internal clock and stimulate your brain.

As you seek to improve the quality of your sleep, you may find it helpful to photocopy or print the recommendations above and read them regularly. If you accidentally omit some of them or have a bad night, don't be discouraged—just get back on track the next day. By following these recommendations over the long haul, you'll establish habits that will promote great sleep opportunities and emotional wellness.

4

REDUCE STRESS

If someone had asked Kelley to describe the last twenty years of her life, two words would have come immediately to her mind: *survival mode*.

Twenty years ago, Kelley was trying to survive an emotionally abusive marriage. When she finally made the decision to leave, she became enmeshed in a grueling and bitter divorce. Then came the financial stress of trying to start a business to support herself and her three children.

Her stress continued to escalate when her ex-husband decided he needed a two-year "break" from paying child support, throwing the family further into financial disarray. Eventually, Kelley hired a family law attorney and took her ex back to court. The judge ruled in her favor, ordering the ex to begin paying child support again and providing reimbursement for the months he didn't pay. Finally caught up on months' worth of overdue bills, Kelley was able to stop foreclosure proceedings on her home with less than a month to spare.

By then, her youngest child was in his midteens and discovering the lure of alcohol. For three frightening years, Kelley lived on high alert as she tried desperately to get her son the help he needed, while navigating the strain of her son's many lies and self-destructive choices.

By the time her youngest came to his senses, committed to sobriety, and was back on the track of becoming a well-adjusted young man, Kelley felt like she was taking her first deep breath in many years.

She was grateful that—finally!—life seemed to have leveled out. Her kids were doing well. She was no longer living paycheck to paycheck. For the first time in a long time, she wasn't waking up in a panic and wondering how she was going to get through the day. Her years of living in survival mode had, at last, come to an end.

Still, Kelley soon realized she had little optimism about the future or enthusiasm for her improved lifestyle. Instead of embracing this new season with joy, Kelley felt herself disengaging from everyone around her. As her isolation grew, she battled increasingly negative thoughts, and her emotions continued their steady decline into what felt like an endless abyss of sadness.

The Science of Stress

The idea that long-term stress and depression are linked goes back many decades. Numerous research studies conclusively demonstrate the detrimental effects of prolonged stress on our emotional and physiological well-being. But you don't need to read medical journals to understand the damaging connection between stress and depression. Certainly, you have seen this dynamic at play in your own life and in the lives of people you love.

There are some commonsense reasons why stress contributes to depression. When we are stressed, we may be tempted to abandon healthy habits we typically follow. Financial stress, for example, can lead to working long hours, skipping exercise, losing sleep due to worry, or eating fast food on the way home from a late night at the office. When we forfeit proper nutrition, exercise, and sleep, we abandon three of our most powerful defenses against depression . . . and we lose three potent coping strategies for managing stress.

What's more, stress can also prompt us to seek temporary relief in unhealthy habits that create *more* stress in the long run. Turning to alcohol, comfort food, or overspending might provide temporary relief and distraction, but these things will complicate our lives and add to our stress over time.

But there's much more to this dynamic than the idea that stress tempts us to abandon good habits and pursue bad ones. Science tells us that when we experience stress—particularly ongoing, chronic stress like Kelley endured—it triggers processes within our bodies that are conducive to depression, even years after the stress or trauma occurred.

The body responds to different threats in different ways. For example, when physical injury or infection has occurred, localized inflammation is the body's signal for help. When skin or tissues are damaged, chemicals are released that increase blood flow to the area and also attract white blood cells to fight pathogens. In other words, inflammation is helping your immune system do its job.

But prolonged stress—especially stress related to interpersonal loss or rejection—triggers something called adaptive immunity, which not only increases inflammation at the sites of past trauma but also increases systemic inflammation throughout the body. And that's where the real problem lies.

Chronic, systemic inflammation has been linked to a variety of serious diseases, including "asthma, arthritis, diabetes, obesity, atherosclerosis, certain cancers, and Alzheimer's disease" . . . and, of course, depression.[1]

Professors at Rice University reviewed two hundred studies on depression and found that depression and inflammation are intertwined, feeding off each other.[2] Furthermore, depression caused by chronic inflammation is resistant to traditional interventions (although it does respond to yoga, biofeedback, meditation, and exercise).

The link between prolonged stress, systemic inflammation, and major depression isn't exactly good news, particularly since the amount of stress we experience today is, according to the American Psychological Association (APA), becoming a public health crisis. In fact, APA CEO Norman Anderson, PhD, says, "America is at a critical crossroads when it comes to stress and our health."[3]

While this is not good news, it does give us a place to begin. It gives us hope that, by managing our stress (and inflammation), we can decrease depression and create a positive difference in our mood.

Take Control of What You Can Control

When our team of experts meets with clients every week, they are reminded that feeling stressed and overwhelmed by the demands of life is a common denominator. Not everything that causes us stress can be eliminated—nor should it. Low-level stress stimulates the brain to boost productivity and concentration. It can also be a big motivator to make changes, solve problems, or accomplish goals that make us better human beings and create improvements in our lives.

In addition, many sources of stress are simply beyond our control. Sometimes things happen that we could not have foreseen or avoided, such as changes in the economy, an employer declaring bankruptcy, an accident or illness, or even other people's decisions that gravely affect us.

That said, there are still plenty of stressors in our lives over which we do have control. Indeed, the elimination of stressors in this category will not only improve our lives but will also leave us healthier and happier. We are often tempted to complain about what we cannot control without ever making an effort to change or manage what we can control.

These controllable factors are the things we ask clients to focus on, and you should focus on them too. Here are six stress-management strategies you should begin practicing immediately.

Stop Procrastinating

This is a simple (though not easy) place to start. It's safe to say we all procrastinate sometimes, and for some people, procrastination is a way of life. Whether you occasionally or serially procrastinate, your delays and avoidance amp up your stress levels. Naturally, the more you procrastinate, the more stressed you become.

Chances are, at this very moment, there is something in your life that is making you feel anxious . . . not because you can't change it but because you are putting off doing what you need to do to resolve that source of stress once and for all. Stop procrastinating, and get that extra stress off your chest.

Limit Your Commitments

Something else that is largely within your control to manage is how overcommitted you are. Granted, sometimes situations impose themselves on our lives and schedules, and we can find ourselves overwhelmed as a result. If we're not careful, we can grow accustomed to the feeling and continue to live in a familiar state of overload by never saying no.

Protecting your time from commitments that are within your control to refuse may not be easy, but it's arguably one of the most effective things you can do to reduce your stress.

Embrace Healthy Escapes

When we're stressed, it's tempting to turn to excessive eating, spending, or alcohol consumption. That's because we want to do something to change our mood! Of course, the list of unhelpful and unhealthy escapes could go on and on. Legal and illegal substance abuse, gambling, pornography, and infidelities may help us temporarily forget about the stress of our lives but will eventually leave us even more stressed—and depressed—than ever.

Being intentional about *how* we escape is critical, and what we choose can determine not only how long we stay stressed but how much damage we sustain in the process.

So what are some examples of healthy escapes? It could be as simple as spending an hour with an enjoyable book in a backyard hammock or as elaborate as planning a trip to a bed-and-breakfast in another state.

You can also take an hour and try something brand new. For example, drive around a part of town you're unacquainted with until you find an unfamiliar coffee shop, go inside, and order something you've never tried before.

Plan a staycation and camp in your backyard. Spend an afternoon at a local zoo or art museum. Visit a tourist attraction in your city that you've never been to before. Taking a walk in nature is an escape that is good for your body, your emotions, and your brain. Watching a favorite comedy is another escape that won't complicate your life or add to your stress after the credits roll.

Finally, you can cultivate healthy habits for when you feel stressed, instead of turning to unhealthy habits (like bingeing on comfort food). One of our clients bought a mini trampoline and placed it near her pantry. Because stress usually turns her toward snacks, she wanted a healthier alternative where she would be sure to see it.

A word of challenge on this point: people who are depressed usually do not want to embrace healthy escapes. They don't feel like it. These pursuits seem pointless or contrived or like too much work. But summon up any energy and motivation you can . . . and just do it!

Put an End to Isolation and Withdrawal

When we're stressed, it's tempting to isolate. When we're already feeling overwhelmed, the last thing we want to do is expend the energy to drive to an event, have someone over, or connect with a friend after work. And yet study after study shows that supportive relationships are huge factors when it comes to improving how we experience and process stress. In fact, loneliness is linked not only to depression but also to health problems including high blood pressure, cardiovascular disease, cancer, and cognitive decline.

It's worth noting here that involvement in a faith community may help in this regard. Studies have shown that people who are involved in faith communities tend to have lower levels of anxiety and stress. People who experience their faith with a supportive community are not only connecting with like-minded people, but they also feel more connected to God. (We'll take a more detailed look at soul care in chapter 7.)

Guard Your Thoughts

Sometimes the source of stress can be found in our own thoughts. Ruminating on negative or painful experiences, refusing to forgive, or practicing a perennially negative outlook on life can create ongoing stress. What's more, because the source of this chronic stress isn't anything external that you can point to, it can be hard to identify and change.

We all have an inner voice constantly blabbering about our faults, failures, inadequacies, and unfortunate experiences. But did you know that you control the on/off switch for that voice? Refuse to sit still for self-inflicted verbal beatings any longer, and dam the flow of negative messages coming into your brain. Replace them with positive affirmations. Accept your shortcomings and celebrate your strengths. Refuse to ruminate about past hurts, and redirect your thoughts to uplifting memories. You will take a big step toward overcoming stress by recognizing the crucial role of thoughts and self-talk in creating your life.

Take Care of Your Body

One of the best things you can do to handle the stresses of life is to fortify your health and body. Eating right, exercising regularly, and getting enough sleep relieve feelings of stress and anxiety, improve your mood, and energize your body, brain, and emotions.

A major study, for example, tracked more than a million individuals to examine the association between exercise and mental health difficulties. Individuals who exercised consistently reported significantly fewer days of poor mental health in the past month than individuals who did not exercise but were otherwise matched for several physical and sociodemographic characteristics. All exercise types were associated with a lower mental health burden.[4]

As I suggested at the outset of this book, many factors cause depression and are interrelated. It's no surprise that taking care of your body through nutrition, exercise, and sleep will not only relieve depression but also aid in reducing stress.

—

It's impossible to eliminate all stress from your life. Managing stress well, thankfully, is another story. How much stress you experience—and how you respond when you experience that stress—is something over which you have more control than you may realize.

By keeping in mind these stress-busting

strategies, you are taking an important step in improving the quality of your life as well as reducing a significant contributor to major depressive disorder.

5

LIMIT TECHNOLOGY USE

Research into the link between technology use and depression is a mixed bag. In some ways, that's to be expected when studying something that's so new. Widespread social media use, for instance, is still not yet two decades old. The hypothesized effects of too much screen time are also largely subjective and difficult to measure. It's hard to get definitive answers when we're still not entirely sure what the right questions are.

Nevertheless, numerous studies point to adverse mental health effects on young people when they spend too much time engaged in online activity. Those include an increase in suicidal thoughts, depression, and anxiety. A University of Pittsburgh School of Medicine study on the effects of social media use, for instance, concluded that "exposure to highly idealized representations of peers on social media elicits feelings of envy and the distorted belief that others lead happier and/or more successful lives"—which can cause depression, the authors wrote.[1]

There is also an unresolved chicken-and-egg dilemma with some research. Studies report a link between internet use and emotional disorders like ADHD, borderline personality disorders, and anxiety, but they often can't reliably pinpoint which came first. In other words, does internet usage impact the onset and severity of mental health issues, or does the presence of those disorders make a person more likely to overuse the internet? These and other questions remain to be answered.

And yet I can confirm from firsthand experience—after working with hundreds of clients over several decades—that the misuse of technology has a direct impact on the severity of depressive symptoms. It's why I have made addressing this behavior a key part of the whole-person approach to conquering depression. When we welcome clients to The Center on their first day, we ask them to relinquish their electronic devices—anything with a screen—for a certain period of time. The reason is simple: to eliminate distractions. We want people to be as present as possible and focused on their recovery process. We store the devices in an office safe for at least seventy-two hours, and in some cases, for the duration of the clients' stay at the clinic.

By the very next day, we notice something remarkable. Most of those people begin to exhibit classic signs of physical withdrawal from an addictive substance. Almost all become irritable and agitated, sometimes developing sweaty palms and an elevated heart rate. Their bodies are responding to the loss of connection via their devices in ways remarkably similar to quitting drugs or alcohol cold turkey. Clearly, something is out of balance in the role technology is playing in their lives.

If we look at the research for a common thread that can help shed light on this experience—and that will suggest ways to alleviate our clients' distress—we find it easily enough. The key lies in the word *misuse* and in how we define it. In other words, technology itself is neither harmful nor beneficial. It's our own choices about how we use technology that will determine our experience.

Hidden Costs

It's not important to decide right now which comes first, digital obsession or emotional depression. What matters is this: if you are already struggling with symptoms of depression, overusing technology can make matters much worse. Here's how.

Addiction

First, some good news: drug, alcohol, and tobacco use among adolescents in the United States has steadily fallen since the 1990s. The bad news? Researchers suspect one reason for that is kids are increasingly substituting technology for these substances as their "drug" of choice. One specialist went so far as to describe the smartphone as "digital heroin" for millennials.[2] That appears to be more than mere hyperbole. Findings suggest the brain reacts similarly to positive feedback on social media, for example, as it does to opioid drugs in the bloodstream.

What's at the heart of any addiction is impulse control—that is, the struggle to say no when faced with a choice that could have negative consequences. For those who are already battling depression, this is a big problem. A common response to the distress of depression is to reach for anything that makes you "feel better." With the world at your fingertips via the internet, the range of self-medication options is practically endless. You are one click away from indulging in impulsive shopping, pornography, and gambling or useless "surfing" or bingeing on entertainment or news. Maybe some or all of that delivers a momentary surge of euphoria . . . with the key word being *momentary.* When it wears off, you want more, and so the cycle of addiction begins.

Of course, as with any addiction, over time the lows grow deeper and the highs not as high, which only reinforces feelings of hopelessness, despair, and worthlessness—all the hallmarks of depression. This is why recovery must include an honest look at the scope of your internet use and treatment for possible addiction to technology alongside everything else.

Isolation

A ubiquitous feature of practically every internet activity is that it's *solitary*. Sure, you may be messaging or chatting or gaming with others who are also online, but generally, you are physically alone. This isolation can be damaging in many ways, but two in particular have negative consequences for people suffering from depression.

First, interacting with others only through electronic media filters our communication and strips away a huge range of important nonverbal signals. Researchers estimate that anywhere from 65 to 85 percent of all communication takes place through eye contact, facial expression, hand gestures, body position and posture, and so on. While we can choose our words carefully—and even use language to say things that are utterly untrue—it's nearly impossible to manipulate our subconscious signals. In other words, most of us tell the truth with body language. If you want to know what a person really thinks and who they really are, you have to be in personal contact with them.

Second, isolation enables us to create false personas—virtual identities that bear little resemblance to who we actually are. These alter egos allow us to adopt traits we ordinarily shun in face-to-face relationships: verbal aggression and overly explicit sexual communications, for example. Or they enable us to hide away all evidence of distress and creeping dysfunction in our real lives.

What a person seeking to heal from depression needs most of all is to focus attention on their life as it really is, to take stock of unhelpful conditions in the real world, and to accept support from real people.

Virtual Conflict

Social isolation and its tendency to enable behavioral extremes is a two-way street. It's damaging to indulge in those things yourself but also to be exposed to them coming from others. Cyberbullying, while normally thought of as a problem only among teens, can happen to anyone online. According to the Pew Research Center, 41 percent of US adults report they've been the target of online harassment, including 18 percent who say the incidents were "severe," such as sustained stalking or threats of violence.[3] Remove the filters and feedback that govern in-person communication and you take away the standards of conduct they are meant to regulate as well.

Here's the bottom line: the last thing a person suffering from depression needs is exposure to a stream of merciless judgments and condemnations masquerading as a chat or a comment. An unhealthy self-image is already a trip wire. Far from diffusing the danger, too much time on the internet is an invitation to make matters worse.

Discomfort with Solitude and Inactivity

A big reason why human beings are drawn to technology is that it stimulates and activates our brains in a way few other things can. The riveting visual imagery, the fast-paced movement of flickering screens, the commotion and constant motion, and the cacophony of noises all get our brain synapses firing at a rapid pace. Overuse of technology often creates a need for more and more stimulation to keep our brains and emotions satisfied. And so we up the ante, seeking additional time with technology and greater intensity from our electronic interactions.

All of this has an often overlooked consequence: a sense of discomfort and restlessness with solitude, stillness, and silence. As a society, we have largely lost appreciation for quietness and introspection. It is in moments of tranquility that we allow our imaginations the freedom to conceive new ideas. It is in moments of contemplation that we listen for spiritual guidance. It is in moments of unhurried reflection that we come to understand who we are as unique individuals.

Technology frequently creates in us a "need for speed," a hunger for nonstop activity and never-ending action. When this occurs, we forfeit the opportunity to grow and to help others grow.

Comparison

It's long been recognized that keeping up with the Joneses is a big part of what keeps us all running the rat race. It's admittedly difficult to avoid noticing the outward appearances of your neighbor's life—job, car, home, overachieving kids, and adventurous vacations—and comparing them to your own, concluding your neighbor must be better off and happier than you. This comparison game is rigged from the start. Media marketers work overtime to be sure you feel your life is lacking so they can sell you what's missing.

Before the internet, however, those we compared ourselves to were mostly flesh-and-blood people. They lived down the street or worked down the hall. It was at least possible to see them at their worst as well as at their best. And they numbered in the dozens at the very most.

Now we compare ourselves to thousands, if not millions, of virtual neighbors. And we see only what they allow us to see—photos of their pets, happy dinners with friends, the view from an exotic beach, kids getting academic awards, crossing the finish line at the Boston Marathon. Most of this is posted by people who are friends in name only. It's a giant understatement to say that all this adds up to a managed and distorted view of who people really are and how they actually live. And that's before we account for perceptions created by advertisers that can be grossly manipulative, misleading, or outright false.

Those suffering from depression are already poised to believe that their lives don't measure up to the lives of others. The internet provides persuasive "evidence" they're right about that.

Toxic Content

While much of what you see on the internet presents an overly rosy view of reality, millions of other sites peddle the opposite extreme: nonstop doom and gloom. It's an alarming parade of war, famine, political strife, social injustice, and environmental catastrophe—almost as if news organizations, bloggers, filmmakers, chat group members, and millions of commenters have conspired to turn whole regions of cyberspace into a scene from Dante's *Inferno*, in which the entrance to hell is inscribed "Abandon hope all ye who enter here!" Spend much time there, and you'll be convinced the world teeters on the edge of calamity and collapse every second of every day.

I believe a steady diet of "digital distortion" is harmful to anyone's mental health and magnifies depression symptoms. It rarely leads to healthy or effective political engagement on important issues. To a person struggling to overcome serious depression, it's positively toxic. Turning off the spigot and cleaning up the digital sludge is an essential step toward recovery.

Physical Stagnation

We've already mentioned that, by definition, most technology use is solitary. Now let's consider the fact that it's also *stationary*. Simple observation will confirm this. A person playing video games will remain in virtually the same position for hours. Someone surfing online will sit hunched over a keyboard, sometimes barely looking up for long periods of time.

Health risks associated with such a sedentary lifestyle are well documented: high blood pressure, heart disease, type 2 diabetes, certain types of cancer, obesity, reduced immune system function—and depression and anxiety.

Limiting Technology Use

There is no need to fear technology in itself. We all know it can be an amazing asset and convenience in our lives. But because of these risk factors, how we use it is of great importance to anyone determined to heal from depression. Finding balance is a checkpoint we can't afford to ignore. Changing your relationship to the internet is a big step on the road to getting there.

Here are six quick ways:

1. Keep an online log to track your digital use for one or two weeks. You can download an app or set your timer to calculate your time spent online. After tracking your daily use for a week or two, you'll have a good idea of how much time you spend connected via the internet. Brace yourself! Most of us underestimate how much time we spend online, similar to alcoholics who underestimate or minimize their alcohol consumption. This exercise is not intended to cause you guilt but to provide a reality check about your technology use.

2. Also track your interaction with other technology. Because of the prevalence of the internet in our society, it gets much of the research attention. But of course that's just one source of technology among many.

Monitor how many hours you spend watching television, playing video games, viewing movies, and so on. Brace yourself again! Adding these hours to your online hours will probably come as a shock.

3. Put yourself on a tech diet. Now that you know your average weekly technology usage, begin to scale back. Start slowly, trimming a half hour from your daily use, then an hour, then more until you achieve a reasonable and comfortable level. The most effective strategy is replacement therapy, meaning you can replace your technology use with enjoyable activities that productively occupy that time: walking with a friend, going to the gym, playing board games with family members, reading a book, tending your garden, or taking up a new hobby.

4. Commit to a periodic digital detox. This means you will set aside a certain period to interact with absolutely no technology. This might be a full day, a weekend, or a week. For many people, this kind of detox will be difficult; for other people, it sounds positively impossible. But it's not only possible; it is also a positive step toward emotional health. Expect plenty of agitation and restlessness. As said earlier, setting aside your devices often causes a sense of withdrawal, akin to drug withdrawal symptoms. Don't dismiss how difficult a digital detox can be—but also how liberating it can be.

5. Curtail social media engagement. Checking Facebook, Instagram, and other sites every other day (or less frequently) should suffice. It's wonderful to keep up with the activities of friends and family members, but let's be honest—most posts and notifications could be skipped without missing anything important. Also, be wary of "friends" who project a perfect, polished online presence. You don't need to view posts that cause you to feel envious or inferior.

6. Keep your device out of the bedroom. As we examined in chapter 3, developing good sleep habits is a key factor in conquering depression. When our phones or other devices are close at hand to where we sleep, it can be tempting to do one last check-in before bed, which can upset the sleep habits you've been trying to cultivate. The best way to resist temptation is to keep your devices away from where you sleep.

6

RELEASE ANGER, FEAR, AND GUILT

In my decades of working with people desperate to overcome depression, I have learned that what I call the three deadly emotions—anger, fear, and guilt—are nearly always present to some degree in the hearts and minds of people suffering from depression. Regardless of what triggers these emotions, anger, fear, and guilt can cause great damage in your life and can hinder your recovery. Here are just a few common sources of toxic anger I've seen:

- mistreatment (real or perceived) during childhood
- being unfairly denied promotion at work or deserved recognition in other contexts
- unresolved conflicts with family and friends
- infidelity and divorce
- illness and the sense of "why me?" injustice it can prompt
- financial misfortune
- grief at a painful loss that turns to bitterness
- general social injustice and "righteous rage"

It's important to notice that everything on this list could just as easily be a source of guilt and fear instead. The interplay between these deadly emotions is like an ever-shifting kaleidoscope, each twisted shape blending into the next. For instance, change the circumstances, and anger at a spouse's infidelity becomes guilt for your own, or fear of possible unfaithfulness in the future. Perhaps anger is followed by the guilty feeling that a partner's infidelity is proof there is something desperately wrong with *you*, leading to the fear that you don't deserve to be happy again.

Can you see why thought patterns like these are so detrimental to your mental health? It is difficult to say which comes first, runaway deadly emotions or depression. But in any case, they have a proven and powerfully negative influence on one another. If you are prone to depression for other reasons, these toxic feelings will rob you of the natural resilience you need to keep or regain your balance.

Here's the important part for anyone struggling with depression: lasting healing is not possible when unexamined and untended anger, guilt, and fear smolder beneath the surface of your life. They will undermine any progress made on other fronts—such as nutrition, sleep, and exercise—and place a hard limit on what's possible. For this reason, while some traditional treatments for depression ignore these emotions, the whole-person model makes diffusing them a high priority, just as important as any other link in the chain of healing.

A Time for Everything

We won't come any closer to healing depression if we simply brand anger, guilt, and fear as undesirable and attempt to bury them away. Like many dangerous things, even emotions that can have such a deadly effect on mental and physical health may also play a positive role in our lives. The trick is in seeing the fundamental difference between the side of our emotions that leads to the darkness of depression and the side that is healthy and life giving.

The key to understanding lies in the word *power*.

The immediate result of runaway and deadly anger, guilt, and fear is not depression; it is a sense of *powerlessness*, the belief that you have no control over the circumstances of your life. This is the soil in which depression grows.

Is it possible for those same emotions to lead to empowerment instead? Yes, it is. In fact, that's the purpose of proper and balanced emotions—even heated ones like anger, guilt, and fear. They are meant to guide us into thoughts and actions that make life better. Here's how.

Anger. There are times when anger is not only appropriate but also positively beneficial. That's because anger—like pain—is a signal that something is not right in our environment. Something important needs our attention. Anger motivates us to

- correct what needs correcting, in the world and in ourselves;
- set and keep personal boundaries;
- defend ourselves when threatened;
- stand up for others in need of help; and
- lend our voices to important issues in our communities.

Appropriate anger is the warning light on the dashboard of our lives alerting us to the need for action.

Guilt. There are two types of guilt—*self-correcting* and *self-loathing*. You might also call them true guilt (justified) and false guilt (unjustified). The first occurs naturally when you recognize you've made a mistake. It's a spontaneous emotional signal that you need to make amends and give thought to avoiding the same mistake in the future.

It's obvious from its name that the second type of guilt—self-loathing—is the kind that contributes to depression. It may also be prompted by a particular incident, but rather than encouraging introspection and self-improvement, it results in a generalized feeling of unworthiness. That's not something we know how to correct, so it lingers and grows until it stops being about something we may have *done* and becomes a statement on *who we are*: worthless. Combine that with other common ingredients and you've got a recipe for depression.

Fear. If you are walking alone through a darkened parking lot at night in a rough neighborhood, a dose of fear-induced adrenaline is a helpful asset. It sharpens your senses and reflexes, preparing you to fight or flee, should it become necessary. It's what kept our ancestors alive back when the "neighborhood" was likely to be filled with hungry carnivores and pillaging enemies.

But what happens when fear (or anger or guilt) becomes a way of life—no longer a momentary response to specific dangers but a constant, low-level tension? In that case, these emotions have exactly the opposite effect, with all sorts of physical and emotional consequences—including depression. According to researchers at Mayo Clinic,

> the long-term activation of the stress-response system—and the subsequent overexposure to cortisol and other stress hormones—can disrupt almost all your body's processes. This puts you at increased risk of numerous health problems, including: anxiety, depression, digestive problems, headaches, heart disease, sleep problems, weight gain, memory and concentration impairment.[1]

Incidentally, the stress-response system surrounding fear releases the same neurochemicals as chronic anger does—adrenaline and cortisol. Research has shown that, while these two compounds are essential and beneficial in short bursts, chronic exposure produces significant disruption to your body's immune system, opening the door to all manner of secondary health problems. One of the most striking things about the list of health problems above is that it's full of conditions that mental-health professionals encounter with people who believe they are simply suffering from depression. In other words, depression never stands alone. It is always both the circular cause and the effect of numerous other factors—including letting the three deadly emotions go unresolved.

The good news is that your emotions do not have to dictate the direction of your life, including your struggle with depression. It is possible to keep your emotions in balance so that they empower you and don't encumber you. You need not live as your emotions' hostage. It is possible to regain the upper hand over what you feel and why.

The Antidote to Toxic Emotion: Forgiveness

There is a proven antidote to toxic emotion—and a powerful tonic for regaining control over your health and well-being. However, like everything else on the road to conquering depression, it's not a magic elixir you can ingest for instantaneous and miraculous relief. This cure will require tough choices, discipline, and commitment on your part. It will take courage to face your emotional dragons and to dare to think differently about them. But it can be done! Proof lies in the millions of people who have gone before you and found freedom in the age-old practice of *forgiveness.*

Now, I am well aware that *forgiveness* is a loaded word for many people. It carries conflicting religious overtones or hints of pop culture sentimentalism many of us have learned to mistrust. For many of us, anger, guilt, and fear are more than mere emotions. They've become an armored identity. We wonder who and what we'll be if we let go.

Well, we'll be better off, that's what—100 percent of the time.

Forgiveness is a blessing, not a burden. It's a source of the very peace you're looking for when pursuing lasting relief from depression. And that's not just wishful thinking. It's amply supported by scientific research.[2]

What Forgiveness Isn't

Before we talk about what forgiveness is, let's examine some misconceptions about forgiveness that keep people stuck in bondage to their angry and fearful judgments.

Forgiveness isn't about letting someone "off the hook." The first and most powerful objection we encounter is the mistaken idea that to forgive means looking the other way while somebody "gets away" with something.

The misunderstanding lies in the belief that forgiving someone is the same thing as excusing the offense. It isn't. In fact, the purpose of forgiveness is not to deliver anything at all to the one who caused us harm but to benefit *ourselves* by letting go of toxic attachment to the past and to our pain. So long as we hang on to feelings of outrage, injustice, and desire for payback, we keep the offense alive and the wounds fresh. And in the process, we remain vulnerable to all the negative physical and psychological effects of runaway anger and fear.

Forgiveness isn't a sign of weakness or an invitation to further offense. This fear appears to be rooted in the ancient human impulse to deal out judgment and retribution for personal or familial offenses. The belief was that if we don't take justice into our own hands, no one else will act on our behalf, leaving the door open for more trespasses of our boundaries.

And yet, ask yourself this: Which is a bigger sign of weakness: letting the offensive actions of someone else determine your future health and well-being, or taking charge of your own destiny by choosing forgiveness over bondage to anger and fantasies of revenge?

Forgiveness isn't the same thing as reconciliation. Most of the time, the goal after a painful conflict with someone we care about is to put the relationship back on track and move ahead with life. This is called reconciliation, a process that can even serve to make us stronger and more tolerant of each other. In the case of most ordinary offenses, this is a good and healthy endeavor. Otherwise, we'd have no relationships at all, since it's impossible to go through life without occasionally stepping on each other's toes.

But while forgiveness is usually a necessary step in reconciliation, the inverse is not true.

Sometimes a person's trespass is so harmful or severe that continuing the relationship is impossible or inadvisable. It's always possible to forgive in such cases, for reasons we've already discussed. But reconciliation is a different matter involving evidence of real remorse, restorative restitution, and future guarantees of safety. When healing from a serious offense, that's a high standard that requires the genuine participation of both parties.

As we employ forgiveness as a tool for healing depression, it's important that you don't confuse the two. If reconciliation is possible, wonderful. You'll find that to be a source of healing as well. But if not, rest assured that forgiveness can still be your powerful ally.

Full-Spectrum Forgiveness

By looking closely at what forgiveness isn't, we've also begun forming a better idea of what it is. Forgiveness is the way to liberate yourself from toxic attachments to old wounds and emotions that are directly responsible for your depression and other ill effects. Step one is accepting that this is true and that your freedom is worth the effort it will take to retrain yourself to let go. If you can get *there* and choose to honestly try forgiveness for a change, then the details of *how* will fall into place.

But first, we need to pick up one last bit of insight for the journey: a look at *all* those in need of your forgiveness. So far, we've talked only of people who have harmed or offended you in some way, and we've seen how an inability to forgive them keeps you enslaved to your pain. But those may not be the only ones against whom you harbor feelings of resentment and judgment.

Forgiving yourself. In many respects, this task is harder than grappling with the offenses of flesh-and-blood others. That's because things we hold against ourselves tend to be internal and unseen, which means larger than life. As we lie awake in the wee hours of the morning, our own perceived offenses grow in our minds to monstrous proportions. They cease being about what we may have done and become damning evidence of who we are—*horrible human beings*. That, you may notice, is often the mind-set of people who suffer from depression, a deeply entrenched belief in their own worthlessness.

It's not true, of course. Take away the word *horrible*, and you've got the truth of it: we're all just human beings, flawed and prone to all kinds of blunders.

Have you made choices you are not proud of? Certainly.

Have you disappointed others who had a right to depend on you? Yes.

How do I know? Because you are human, and every human on earth is a combination of strengths and weaknesses, assets and liabilities, successes and failures.

The irony is that we typically hold ourselves to a standard that's much higher than what we expect of others. It's an inverted kind of arrogance that causes us to set up a wall of shame in our minds, where all our flaws, large and small, are on display under bright light.

Here's the key to forgiveness when you're the one on trial: visualize yourself in court, but not as you appear today. See yourself as a child of six or seven. How would that child feel? Frightened? Alone? In need of comfort? Imagine taking a seat beside your small self and saying, "It's okay. You're learning. You'll be a better person because of this experience." This is how to defeat the second of the three deadly emotions, guilt: by forgiving yourself.

Forgiving God. Whom do we blame for painful events that seem to come out of nowhere, beyond anyone's control? We blame

God, of course—or "life"—for being cruel and unfair. Theologians and philosophers have wrestled for centuries with the question of why such things happen, and none has produced a universally satisfactory answer. We're simply left with a hard truth: bad things happen, and most of the time there's little or nothing to be done about it. Sometimes those events are unspeakably painful, and the temptation to give up on the very idea of a loving and omnipotent God is immense.

Yet clinging to universal resentment at "the way things are" is only a recipe for making your experience of them worse. Again, it is not necessary to say "It's okay" about something that clearly isn't. But it's also not okay to enslave yourself to misery by refusing to let go of your anger and pain. The key is in letting go of the need for explanations. Chances are you'll never know why certain things happen . . . but you can know *peace* in spite of the unknowns.

Start Today

You are your own greatest ally and asset in your quest to conquer depression. That's because forgiveness will enable you to take a giant step toward wholeness, and forgiveness is something that can only happen within yourself. Far from being an abstract religious concept, deciding to follow God's urging to practice forgiveness is powerful progress in your journey back to wellness.

As I've pointed out, numerous studies have identified a strong link between forgiveness and depression recovery. Even so, you might still be tempted to say, "That's all well and good for others, but I'm just not a very forgiving person."

There's good news for you too. Those same studies have revealed that the ability to forgive can be *learned.* Here are several ways to make forgiveness part of your recovery:

1. Make a clear choice. If you've harbored resentment against someone for a long time, your mind will resist attempts to reverse direction and forgive. To signal that you are serious about getting free, create a contract with yourself. Write, "I hereby pledge to forgive for the following offenses and for the following reasons." Be specific. Argue the case for why forgiveness is the right choice. Sign and date it, then put it somewhere you can easily reach when you need it.

2. Practice empathy. It's important to think of those who have hurt you as ordinary human beings, not monsters. Every human act—even horrific ones—springs from a person's own toxic mix of anger, guilt, fear, and woundedness. While this does not excuse a person's bad behavior, it is an exercise in finding a reason for compassion. From there, it's much easier to contemplate forgiving them and moving on.

3. Employ gratitude. There are few things more powerful than listing all the things you are grateful for in your life. Write them down, say them out loud, and shout them if you can. Do this sincerely and consistently, and you'll soon realize your anger and pain at the unforgiven offense is not so hot or heavy as it was. That's because it's impossible to think two thoughts at once. You can't be grateful and harbor fantasies of revenge at the same time.

4. Dwell in the present. Any offense you have not yet forgiven only exists in the past. The thief is not continuously breaking into your house; your friend's betrayal only happened once. To stop reliving such events over and over, center your thoughts in the safety of here and now. Many techniques exist for doing this. Find one that works for you and give it a try.

5. Ask God for help. Forgiveness does not come naturally to us in the wake of a painful trauma or offense. We must learn how to do it. We must learn how to truly *mean* it. Fortunately, the Great Teacher, our gracious heavenly Father, is ready to show us the way—when we ask.

7

PRACTICE SOUL CARE

In the early 1980s, I had already launched The Center: A Place of Hope. The effectiveness of our work with those who were struggling with eating disorders had drawn broad attention, and my team and I had begun to develop the "whole person" model for helping people heal after other methods had fallen short. More and more desperate individuals came to our clinic; media opportunities became frequent; speaking engagements and consultations crowded my calendar. I was busy advising others on how to take charge of their overall health and lifestyle habits to achieve the change they so badly wanted in their lives and was seeing real, tangible results.

All the while my own life was rapidly falling apart.

Working six days a week at a grueling (and foolish) pace, I had begun to make the classic mistake of not practicing what I preached. My diet was a wreck, and I made no attempt to exercise. I self-medicated with false comforts like junk food, excessive caffeine, and other unhealthy choices. Nighttime became a nightmare of insomnia and anxiety. Days were not much better. A deep emotional apathy and physical lethargy overtook my waking hours. I gained weight and looked haggard. Depleted and desperate, I was not much better off than many of my patients.

After months of this downward spiral, something happened that turned my life around—without which I honestly don't know where I'd be today.

My lifeline came, ironically enough, in the form of total exhaustion. The people who cared about me most—family members and close friends—stepped in and stepped up to steer me back on course, demonstrating equal measures of loving support and tough love. They worked to put me on a rigidly controlled daily routine that reinstated the healthy habits I knew but wasn't practicing. This involved shortened workdays, regular walks, improved sleep habits, a nutritious diet, time for prayer and reflection, and much more. I had to set new boundaries, and I committed to staying within them, and so I began my long climb back to health and well-being.

This is the story I often tell about my own struggle with depression, and it's not unusual when I tell that story in group settings for someone to approach me afterward, still unsatisfied. They sense something is missing from my account because it sounds too simple, too formulaic.

"My family has tried everything yours did," one woman suffering from depression told me. "It's never enough. What made you so different?"

The only honest answer is *absolutely nothing*. I am no different, and certainly no better, than anyone else alive. Yet the question brings up an important point. While there is nothing special about *me*, there was (and still is) something present in my life that played a powerful role in my recovery.

In a word: faith.

I grew up among devout Christian family members. Some of my earliest and fondest memories are set in church gatherings, surrounded by a community of people who had decided to give their lives to God. So when, later in life, I faced my own struggle with depression, there was a dormant X factor buried in my heart and mind that, in the end, made all the difference. While at the time my spiritual life felt like just another obligation, it's also true that the loving intervention of my family and friends might not have been enough if I hadn't also learned the instinct to cry out to God with a single, simple plea: Help!

Now, faith comes in many forms, and God can be found in many places. What follows is the road map and key landmarks I've drawn from my own Christian journey that helped in my own recovery. My goal is not to impose my beliefs on you. Rather, these are practices drawn from my experience of faith that have proved to be effective spiritual tools for me and those we serve at The Center, and my prayer is that they will help you to care for your soul as you seek to conquer depression.

Choose to Have Faith

In times of crisis, when well-meaning people advise you to "have faith," they often make it sound simple, as if it's possible to magically "have" something as elusive as faith on command. That's nearly as unhelpful as telling someone who's suffering from depression to simply "feel better." Every step on the path to recovery requires courage and commitment, all summed up in one powerful word: *choice*. You must choose to seek help and choose to pursue the remedies you are offered before you can tap into their healing potential.

Faith is no different. It's not an ethereal "thing" we try to grasp; it's more like an action—something we do on purpose. True, God is willing and able to meet you exactly where you are and to carry you for as long as it takes to restore your strength. In fact, I believe it would astonish us to see how often we benefit from God's unseen work around us. But faith is our part to play to actively complete the circuit of God's love. We do that by choosing to believe we are not alone—through sheer force of will, if necessary—when the night is at its darkest. *God* does not need our faith; *we* do. His strength does not wane; ours does.

Faith, precisely because it begins with a determined choice, is a jolt of energy that activates our spiritual and emotional immune system as nothing else can. How? By opening the door to the one thing that all people who suffer from depression feel they have lost forever: hope. As the writer of the book of Hebrews assures us, "Faith is confidence in what we hope for and assurance about what we do not see" (11:1).

That writer knew what it meant to hope for something we can't yet see, and he understood that active, determined faith sustains us while we wait for the thing we want to materialize and work to make it so. We might face a health crisis, financial problems, relationship strain, or job loss. Not every hardship we endure will turn out exactly the way we want, but we have the assurance that these things will ultimately result according to God's will and God's best for us. We have this confidence because our faith does not rest in fate or chance or any other thing on earth. Our faith is in God, who is unfailingly good.

One way or another, you always choose how to face your life, with confidence or with doubt, in strength or in defeat. Given those options, why not choose the power of faith?

Talk to God

Another way to care for your soul is to talk to God. You might be wondering, *Don't you mean "pray"?* That depends on your definition of that often-misunderstood word. If by pray you mean "mutter a stream of rote, repetitious phrases you once heard in church"—things you'd never say to an intimate friend—then, no, that's definitely not what I mean. If prayer, to you, typically consists of a dreary session of complaining and self-condemning, that's also not what I have in mind.

Here's the point: the hope that's restored when you choose faith over despair is *real.* It's the priceless assurance that you are loved—beyond all reason—by a Creator who never takes his eyes off you for a second. He's the type who gleefully gets out his wallet to show off photos of all his children to anyone nearby.

What would you tell *that* person over a cup of tea today? Where it hurts? Your small (and large) victories? Your dreams and ambitions? Maybe your nightmares and disappointments? Would you ask some tough questions? Tell him what you fear? What you love? What you want? Would you laugh and cry together?

I believe you would. And you can. A heartfelt and honest conversation with God is yours for the having. Perhaps best of all, when talking with God, you can ask for wisdom and guidance amid all your struggles. Everyone on earth could use divine direction and understanding in their daily lives, and this is especially true for those battling depression. Prayer is a powerful source of insight and inspiration as you pursue healing.

Listen Closely

Many people scoff at the idea that God speaks back but only because they've never heard an audible voice answer them directly. A key word when we think about prayer is *conversation*—two-way communication. Why bother to pray if we have no hope of receiving a reply? The truth is, God speaks all the time, and we would have no trouble hearing him if we'd only broaden our definition of speech. The psalmist wrote,

> The heavens declare the glory of God;
> the skies proclaim the work of his
> hands.
> Day after day they pour forth speech;
> night after night they reveal knowledge.

> They have no speech, they use no words;
> no sound is heard from them.
> Yet their voice goes out into all the earth,
> their words to the ends of the world.
>
> PSALM 19:1-4

As this psalm so eloquently describes, God certainly speaks through nature. That message is one of majesty and grandeur, to be sure, but also of balance, beauty, and rebirth—qualities we can cling to in tough times.

That's just the beginning. Because God is the Creator, his voice can be heard all over his creation. God's voice can be heard in art and music and stories that inspire us to be more and do better. He speaks in every act of kindness, no matter how small. God's part of the conversation is found in sacred Scriptures and in the words of wise people throughout time who have labored to bring light into the darkness of ignorance. God speaks in our dreams and in subtle moments of intuition.

But as in every conversation, it's possible not to hear a word of it. Why? Because we're not listening. Until we choose to believe God will actually answer our questions and calm our fears, we may frantically do all the talking and never make room for his reply. To avoid this unnecessary mistake, we must slow down, set aside time to be quiet, and extend our awareness. If we go looking for the diverse love notes from God that litter the world, we will find them.

Cultivate Gratitude

Simply put, gratitude fosters optimism, which strengthens hope. That's why it's hard to imagine a more effective soul medicine than gratitude. The list of things we can and should be thankful for, even in our darkest moments, is practically inexhaustible.

Sometimes severe depression makes it hard to muster gratitude for the big things like being alive or the loved ones in your life. So start with the little ones. Anyone can come up with those—the more whimsical, the better.

For example, I'm grateful for ice cream and for the inspired genius who invented it. I'm glad that freshly mowed grass is part of my world on summer evenings, how it smells and how it feels on bare feet. How about you?

Try saying thank you—out loud and with gusto—for teriyaki sauce or butterflies or kites or Mozart . . . anything that has ever made you smile. Say thank you for hot showers and soft towels. Roller coasters. Baseball. Elvis Presley. Fireworks. Tulips poking out of the dirt. A child's unrestrained giggle. That magic moment when the lights go down in the movie theater.

Gratitude is a multiplier, not of the beauty and good all around us in the world, but of our *awareness* of it. And gratitude also makes us more aware of the loving God responsible for it all. When dark thoughts threaten to push everything else aside, purposeful gratitude to our Creator is a powerful way to push back.

Come Clean about Your Mistakes

Even as a kid, I learned it was incredibly liberating to own up to something I'd done that I was not proud of. Trying to keep a dark secret from my parents, a teacher, or a friend was exhausting, like walking around with my pockets full of rocks. The moment I told the truth, it was as if the lights came on and all that weight disappeared. Even if there were still consequences to face, I learned that I always felt better to have the truth out in the open.

That is what the concept of confession is all about—setting us free from the dread of discovery when we're in the wrong. Like the active choice to have faith, this is not for

God's benefit but for ours. Taking responsibility serves as a powerful reminder that we're only human after all. That is paradoxically empowering. Fear of exposure arises in part from the misguided belief that we ought to be more than we are, when the fact is God expects no such thing. The moment we admit our frailties, we find the strength and the motivation to be and do better in the future. Confession compels us to acknowledge who we are and to continually seek to improve.

What's more, confession puts us in the position to receive God's peace, comfort, and forgiveness. *Confess* has its origin in "agreement." So beyond the relief from worrying that we might be found out, confession means agreeing with God about our wrongdoing—and then agreeing with him in how we might work to make it right. The psalmist provides insight into the healing process: "When I kept silent, my bones wasted away through my groaning all day long. . . .

Then I acknowledged my sin to you and did not cover up my iniquity. I said, 'I will confess my transgressions to the LORD.' And you forgave the guilt of my sin" (Psalm 32:3, 5).

Gather Together

One of the most formidable enemies facing people working to heal from depression is *isolation*. By ourselves, we're far more likely to get stuck in unhealthy habits and distorted thought patterns. Our lives become closed echo chambers endlessly reinforcing our sense of hopelessness and despair. What's needed to break through those lonely walls is a community of caring people willing to open their arms and make room for one more fellow traveler.

The right faith community can be just that. Most of my fellow Christians have come to their faith by one difficult road or another. People who share your faith will likely understand the challenges you face in your journey back from depression because they've walked a similar path. They'll provide a nonjudgmental shoulder to lean on.

Belonging to a faith community also provides a tangible reminder that you are not the only struggling person in the world. There's healing in remembering that life does not revolve around you and that even in your darkest moments, you are not uniquely alone. Furthermore, church gatherings will reveal that music, celebration, joy, gratitude, and service are all still alive and well in the world. A dozen or a hundred or a thousand voices all singing together can be an effective salve to a wounded heart.

Serve

Once you see you're not alone in your struggles, the next step is to make a difference in someone else's life. Faith communities usually excel at providing volunteer opportunities and steering you to the one that's right for you.

But even if involvement in a faith community is not your thing, you can find ample ways to be of use to your community if you look for them. Every major city in America has homeless shelters, counseling centers for victims of domestic violence, animal rescue organizations, wounded veterans programs, hospice centers, cancer support groups, suicide prevention clinics, nursing homes filled with people in need of a friend—the list could go on for pages. All of these programs depend on volunteers who know what it's like to need a boost. Best of all, the benefit of service is a two-way street, making life better for you as well as for those you help. A 2007 paper published by the Corporation for National and Community Service called *The Health Benefits of Volunteering* states, "Volunteer activities can strengthen the social ties that protect individuals from isolation during difficult times, while the experience of helping others leads to a sense of greater self-worth and trust."[1]

One study cited in the report concluded that people who volunteer in service to others live longer than those who don't.[2] Think of it this way: by getting involved in church outreach in your community, or by volunteering on your own, you essentially write yourself a prescription for relief from your troubles—free of charge!

—

In my own battle with depression, my faith proved instrumental in bringing me through the darkness. As you consider what "whole person" healing looks like for you, do not neglect these soul care practices. Our selves are a unified whole of body, mind, and spirit, and our healing will not be complete without addressing each aspect of ourselves.

CONCLUSION

REINVENT YOUR FUTURE

By the time Stephanie came to me, depression had upended every area of her life to the point of near complete dysfunction. Just twenty-nine years old, she was a chain-smoker and drank an average of ten liters of caffeinated soda every day. She slept no more than a few hours a day and spent the other groggy twenty-one hours channel surfing between cable news programs. No frightening or ugly thing could happen in the world without Stephanie's knowledge.

After many disappointing attempts at

intervention, her parents and siblings had all but given up on her. She would listen politely, concede that her life was a wreck, and then do nothing. Not surprisingly, she seemed ready to give up on herself—almost. Grasping one last time at frail hope, she agreed to our help.

The next few weeks proved one thing beyond any doubt: Stephanie was a fighter. After a predictably rough start, she muscled her way through everything my staff and I challenged her to do. As she began to emerge from the fog of exhaustion, poor nutrition, substance abuse, and toxic thoughts and emotions, Stephanie felt better than she had in years. That sensation multiplied her motivation to succeed. And so she did. There was more work to do, but she had successfully torn out the old, crumbling foundation of her life and laid a new one, ready to start rebuilding.

And yet, just before leaving our clinic for home, Stephanie approached me with a look of panic on her face. She came to my office to talk, and the reason for her distress poured out in a confused tangle.

"I have no idea what comes next," she said, on the verge of tears. "For so long, just getting back to normal seemed impossible. Now I realize, I don't know what else to hope for!"

Stephanie expressed a common fear among people coming out of a lengthy bout with depression. It is summed up in the question *Now what?* After months or years of barely getting through the day, achieving more than that feels like an unreachable fantasy—even after the fog has lifted.

I'm happy to tell you it's no fantasy! You haven't fought this hard and come this far just to plod through a mediocre life. An *extraordinary* future is now yours for the taking. You're free—not just from depression but free to succeed, to grow, to have adventures, to meet new people, to learn new things, to experience new reasons to love life. In other words, you are just like everyone else—empowered to have your life the way you want it. Here's how.

Reclaim Your Desires

It's remarkable how often people have trouble finishing the simple sentence "I want . . ." I don't mean lofty, beauty pageant answers like "world peace" or vengeful ones such as "I want my sister to suffer for her cruelty!" I'm talking about the ability to express our basic needs and desires. Somehow the process of growing up teaches most of us to think of what we want out of life as secondary to . . . well, just about everything and everyone else.

Sure, there's a time to work hard and sacrifice short-term satisfaction for our goals. But when that becomes all there is to living, problems arise. Desire is the fuel that powers achievement. Without it, there's a hard limit to what you will even try.

To test yourself for a lost connection to your desires, take out a piece of paper and write, "I want." Now make a list of all the ways you might answer the question. The only rule is you can't write something that's for someone else. Each item must reflect something you want for yourself. The desires can be practical ("I want a car that starts every time I turn the key") or more extravagant ("I want the beachside vacation I've dreamed of for years"). Don't overthink your desires—let them flow. Don't stop until you've listed at least twenty.

Now consider: Does this exercise make you uncomfortable? Do you find yourself thinking you don't deserve the things you've placed on the list? Is there a part of you that scoffs, *Yeah right, like* that's *ever going to happen*? Do you worry what others would think if you suddenly indulged yourself by pursuing something on the list? Does your memory replay for you all the bad things that happened the last time you dared to say, "I want . . ." and acted on your desire?

If you answered yes to any of these questions, then it's likely depression has stolen your desires from you—and it's time to take them back.

Begin by looking again at your list. How many of the items express things that you once loved but stopped doing for one reason or another? Drawing? Sailing? Cooking? Cross-country motorcycle riding? Writing a novel that is now half finished and gathering dust in the closet? Working at a job that gave you great satisfaction but little money?

Reclaiming your desires is really about remembering what you *love*. When you were a kid, nobody could stop you from doing cartwheels on the lawn, searching for arrowheads in the vacant lot down the street, reading comic books by the dozen, jumping off the high diving board once you learned you could—because you loved it.

Contrary to what you may believe, that kind of carefree passion is not just for kids. What a bleak world that would be! Fortunately, that's not the world as it really is.

Give yourself permission to want and reach for your desires, and the future will light up in front of you. Getting back in touch with your wants and wishes will empower you to dream again. With renewed knowledge of what brings you joy and rekindled optimism for the future, you can do away with limiting, sabotaging thoughts and revive an old dream that you abandoned . . . or create a big, bold, new one.

Reboot Your Imagination

Here's a startling truth: *everything* ever created by human beings—from the first stone wheel to the International Space Station orbiting the earth today—began as a vision located exclusively in someone's mind. In other words, before we create anything, we must first *see* it. Go ahead and test that claim for yourself. Try to fold a paper airplane without visualizing its finished shape first. Or draw a picture of a rose, but don't imagine how you'll shape the petals or what color you'll choose. It's not just difficult; it's impossible. We are made to imagine, and the world is made of our imaginings.

Here's the point: in the depths of depression, your imagination was hijacked and habituated to project only dull, dark, and dreary outcomes. That state of mind imagines worst-case scenarios. It projects hardship and lack everywhere it looks. And since seeing is the precursor to creating, is it any surprise that this is the vision the world reflected back to you?

To build a brighter future, begin by imagining—in vivid detail—exactly what you want it to look like. In contrast to your former habits, refuse to imagine anything that might go wrong. You get to choose what you see, after all. Do you want genuine romance in your life? Picture your dream partner as clearly as you can. Imagine yourself with this person, in love and fulfilled. Include laughter, affection, adventure—all the things you want in a relationship. Not only will your moment-to-moment experience of life improve when your thoughts are filled with hopeful images, but you can also rest assured that unseen cogs are shifting into place to bring your vision out of your head and into the world.

The practice of picturing what you want works with anything at all: a better job, a new home, improved health, closer relationships, or anything else. That's because you'll set about creating what you envision. Every time. But the true power lies in making an ally out of your imagination where it really counts: *how you see yourself.* Replace the distorted self-image you created when depressed with a new one that's happy, healthy, powerful, prosperous, and free.

Revive Your Purpose

Many people hear the word *purpose* and think it applies only to epic, world-changing work. Not so. I define purpose as the *one unique thing* we each have to offer the world, no matter how big or small. Its absence might not make headlines, but it absolutely would be missed by those who stand to benefit from your gifts. Your personal purpose may be to pour all your energy and creativity into raising healthy children; to teach watercolor painting to residents in a retirement center; to be the most caring and conscientious insurance agent your clients have ever known; or to teach preschool in a way that endows kids with self-respect and self-confidence. The list of possibilities is infinite. Only you can know which one best describes you.

Here's the secret to finding your purpose: start by looking again at the list you made of things you have loved in your life. Chances are, what you're meant to do now is something you couldn't stop doing as a younger person but that you abandoned along the way. Or it may be the thing you still didn't dare put on the list but that tugs at your sleeve anyway.

Why is finding and following your purpose so important when revitalizing your future? Because it's what gets you out of bed on a dreary Monday morning in midwinter. Purpose is your answer to the question "Why?" Why keep a grip on my addictive impulses? Why watch what I eat? Why care about toxic emotions and their effect on my health and well-being? Why guard against old habits?

Because you have a purpose, a role to play in the lives of others. Those others may be abandoned animals at the local shelter or everyone who looks at a piece of your art and is inspired or moved. It may be cliché these days, but it's never been more true:

the world needs *everyone* to fulfill their purpose—you included.

Recover Your Joy

It's safe to say that one thing you forgot through your struggle with depression is how to have *fun*. Admit it: some party-pooper part of you just rolled its eyes and mumbled that "fun" is for other people. The best you can hope for, you think, is not to be disappointed.

I know, because that's how I felt after months of having all my senses—including my sense of humor—bleached and hung out to dry by depression. It was as if the candy was stripped out of life and only a dry mouthful of cotton was left. Live like that for very long, and the words *pleasure* and *enjoyment* start to sound like a foreign language.

But it's instructive to notice that the word *enjoyment* means "the process of taking pleasure in something." *Process. Taking.* These are active words, things we purposely do and participate in. You can sit and wait for joy to strike spontaneously, and it sometimes does. But why would you want to when it's possible to make it happen for yourself? As with so many other things we've discussed, the power of enjoyment is triggered by choice.

Start by silencing your inner critic, who pronounces judgment on every possible source of fun . . . before you even try it! A rafting excursion? Too wet, too dangerous. A salsa dance class with friends? Too embarrassing. A day at the amusement park? Too childish, too expensive, too loud, too many lines. The good news is, it's possible to displace objections like these with a determined decision to just do it. Will this test the boundaries of your comfort zone? Of course. That's what makes it fun!

Next, make room for humor and lightheartedness all through your day. Turn off the news and start a romantic comedy movie marathon or binge on old sitcom episodes or performances by stand-up comedians. Spend time around people who make you laugh and push you to lighten up. Make it your mission to laugh and smile so readily that people begin to wonder what you know that they don't.

Refuse to Retreat

Your life is a story. Like all stories, yours involves a hero (you), a journey (the battles you've fought), and a prize (lifelong wellness). In fact, that progression is found in every great story ever told, from ancient myths sung by firelight, to fairy tales, to modern blockbuster films. Embedded in all these stories is a blueprint for human progress. In other words, struggling is not failure; it's part of being human. It's how we change and grow stronger.

That's great news. It means you need not

look back on depression with regret but rather with hope that you've survived the ordeal in order to be stronger and better than ever.

But there is another universal truth about heroes you need to know as you look ahead to the rest of your life. True heroes—the ones we love most when we find them in books and movies and real-life stories—are never content to passively let events happen to them. They are the ones who, when things look darkest and all hope seems lost, refuse to give up or give in. They are tenacious beyond all reason. They stubbornly believe in what others say is impossible. They get back up again and again when knocked down.

Now that you've fought your way to the treasure of wellness on your own journey, it's important to dig in your heels and tap into the heroic determination to never, ever give it back. The future is yours. Defend it. Fight for it like the heroes you admire most in your favorite stories.

—

There is nothing more exciting than realizing that the rest of your life can be what you choose to make it. Yes, unforeseen challenges will always be part of the fabric of life. But those need not have the final say in how you experience the world.

My prayer for you is that after reading this book, you have hope that conquering depression is possible. And not only is healing possible, but also, on the other side of depression, a thriving future awaits you.

Depression doesn't have to define your story. You can reinvent your future. Start today!

Appendix

Recommended Resources

Books on Nutrition and Depression

21 Days to Eating Better: A Proven Plan for Beginning New Habits by Gregory L. Jantz (Zondervan, 1998).

The Body God Designed: How to Love the Body You've Got While You Get the Body You Want by Gregory L. Jantz (Strang, 2007).

Breakthrough Depression Solution: Mastering Your Mood with Nutrition, Diet and Supplementation by James M. Greenblatt (Sunrise River Press, 2016).

Happy Gut: The Cleansing Program to Help You Lose Weight, Gain Energy, and Eliminate Pain by Vincent Pedre (HarperCollins, 2015).

The Microbiome Diet: The Scientifically Proven Way to Restore Your Gut Health and Achieve Permanent Weight Loss by Raphael Kellman (Da Capo Lifelong Books, 2014).

The Microbiome Solution: A Radical New Way to Heal Your Body from the Inside Out by Robynne Chutkan (Avery Books, 2015).

The Psychobiotic Revolution: Mood, Food, and the New Science of the Gut-Brain Connection by Scott C. Anderson with John F. Cryan and Ted Dinan (National Geographic, 2017).

The UltraMind Solution: The Simple Way to Defeat Depression, Overcome Anxiety, and Sharpen Your Mind by Mark Hyman (Scribner, 2009).

Books on Exercise and Depression

8 Keys to Mental Health through Exercise by Christina G. Hibbert (W. W. Norton, 2016).

Exercise for Mood and Anxiety: Proven Strategies for Overcoming Depression and Enhancing Well-Being by Michael W. Otto and Jasper A. J. Smits (Oxford University Press, 2011).

Spark: The Revolutionary New Science of Exercise and the Brain by John J. Ratey with Eric Hagerman (Little, Brown, 2013).

Books on Emotional Health and Depression

Anatomy of an Epidemic: Magic Bullets, Psychiatric Drugs, and the Astonishing Rise of Mental Illness in America by Robert Whitaker (Broadway Books, 2015).

Controlling Your Anger before It Controls You: A Guide for Women by Gregory L. Jantz with Ann McMurray (Revell, 2013).

Depression Sourcebook, edited by Keith Jones, Health Reference Series (Omnigraphics, 2017).

Happy for the Rest of Your Life: Four Steps to Contentment, Hope, and Joy—and Three Keys to Staying There by Gregory L. Jantz with Ann McMurray (Siloam, 2009).

Healing the Scars of Childhood Abuse: Moving beyond the Past into a Healthy Future by Gregory L. Jantz with Ann McMurray (Revell, 2017).

How to De-Stress Your Life by Gregory L. Jantz (Revell, 1998).

The Anxiety Reset by Gregory L. Jantz (Tyndale, 2021).

Self-Coaching: The Powerful Program to Beat Anxiety and Depression by Joseph J. Luciani (John Wiley & Sons, Inc., 2007).

Uncovering Happiness: Overcoming Depression with Mindfulness and Self-Compassion by Elisha Goldstein (Atria Books, 2015).

The Upward Spiral: Using Neuroscience to Reverse the Course of Depression, One Small Change at a Time by Alex Korb (New Harbinger Publications, 2015).

Books on Spirituality and Depression

The Blessing: Giving the Gift of Unconditional Love and Acceptance by John Trent and Gary Smalley (Thomas Nelson, 2004).

How to Forgive . . . When You Don't Feel Like It by June Hunt (Harvest House, 2015).

The Inner Voice of Love: A Journey through Anguish to Freedom by Henri J. M. Nouwen (Image Books, 1999).

Jesus Wept: When Faith and Depression Meet by Barbara C. Crafton (Jossey-Bass, 2009).

Unshakable Hope: Building Our Lives on the Promises of God by Max Lucado (Thomas Nelson, 2018).

Books on Technology and Depression

12 Ways Your Phone Is Changing You by Tony Reinke (Crossway, 2017).

Alone Together: Why We Expect More from Technology and Less from Each Other by Sherry Turkle (Basic Books, 2011).

#Hooked: The Pitfalls of Media, Technology, and Social Networking by Gregory L.

Jantz with Ann McMurray (Siloam, 2012).

iDisorder: Understanding Our Obsession with Technology and Overcoming Its Hold on Us by Larry Rosen (Palgrave Macmillan, 2012).

iGen: Why Today's Super-Connected Kids Are Growing Up Less Rebellious, More Tolerant, Less Happy—and Completely Unprepared for Adulthood by Jean M. Twenge (Atria Books, 2017).

Irresistible: The Rise of Addictive Technology and the Business of Keeping Us Hooked by Adam Alter (Penguin Books, 2018).

Rewired: Understanding the iGeneration and the Way They Learn by Larry D. Rosen with L. Mark Carrier and Nancy A. Cheever (Palgrave Macmillan, 2010).

Books on Addiction and Depression

Don't Call It Love: Breaking the Cycle of Relationship Dependency by Gregory L. Jantz and Tim Clinton with Ann McMurray (Revell, 2015).

Food Junkies: The Truth about Food Addiction by Vera Tarman with Philip Werdell (Dundurn Press, 2014).

Healing the Scars of Addiction: Reclaiming Your Life and Moving into a Healthy Future by Gregory L. Jantz with Ann McMurray (Revell, 2018).

Organizations Offering Help for Depression and Mental Health

American Association of Christian Counselors. www.aacc.net. AACC assists Christian counselors, licensed professionals, pastors, and lay church members.

American Psychological Association. www.apa.org. The largest association of psychologists in the world, the APA offers access to the latest information on depression and related conditions like ADHD, eating disorders, and suicide.

Anxiety and Depression Association of America. www.adaa.org. This organization provides detailed facts about various conditions, including depression and its symptoms.

Brain and Behavior Research Foundation. www.bbrfoundation.org. This site provides information about depression, anxiety, and other related conditions. The foundation provides support for research into depression and related conditions.

Depression and Bipolar Support Alliance. www.dbsalliance.org. This is a self-help organization for patients and family members, providing significant information on depression as well as anxiety and bipolar disorder.

Mental Health America. www.mentalhealthamerica.net. This is one of the foremost nonprofit organizations in the mental health field, providing up-to-date news and information.

National Alliance on Mental Illness. www.nami.org. This organization provides education and support pertaining to a wide variety of mental health conditions.

National Institute of Mental Health. www.nimh.nih.gov. As the country's largest organization focusing on mental health conditions, NIMH publishes detailed information about the latest findings on depression, anxiety, ADHD, OCD, and related conditions.

Notes

INTRODUCTION: FIND A NEW PATH FORWARD

1. "Major Depression," National Institute of Mental Health, updated November 2017, https://www.nimh.nih.gov/health/statistics/major-depression.shtml.
2. A summary of research findings can be accessed at Seth J. Gillihan, "What Is the Best Way to Treat Depression?," *Psychology Today*, May 30, 2017, https://www.psychologytoday.com/us/blog/think-act-be/201705/what-is-the-best-way-treat-depression. Also see P. Cuijpers et al., "A Meta-analysis of Cognitive-Behavioural Therapy for Adult Depression, Alone and In Comparison with Other Treatments," *Canadian Journal of Psychiatry* 58, no. 7 (July 2013): 376–85, https://www.ncbi.nlm.nih.gov/pubmed/23870719; S. M. de Maat et al., "Relative Efficacy of Psychotherapy and Combined Therapy in the Treatment of Depression: A Meta-analysis," *European Psychiatry* 22, no. 1 (January 2007): 1–8, https://www.ncbi.nlm.nih.gov/pubmed/17194571.

3. "Depression Basics," National Institute of Mental Health, revised 2016, https://www.nimh.nih.gov/health/publications/depression/index.shtml.
4. Kashmira Gander, "Depression Is a Potential Side Effect of Over 200 Common Prescription Drugs, Scientists Warn," *Newsweek*, June 13, 2018, https://www.newsweek.com/depression-potential-side-effect-over-200-common-prescription-drugs-scientists-974358.

CHAPTER 1: EAT AND DRINK WHAT IS GOOD

1. In this chapter, I focus primarily on nutrition—how the food and drink we consume can have a huge impact on our mental health. But prebiotics, probiotics, and micronutrients (as well as removing toxins from your body) are also part of this larger discussion. For more on this emerging field of research and how it relates to depression, see chapters 11–13 of my book *Healing Depression for Life* (Carol Stream, IL: Tyndale, 2019).
2. Some of this content is adapted from "Depression and Diet," WebMD, updated October 16, 2018, https://www.webmd.com/depression/guide/diet-recovery#1.
3. See Kathleen M. Zelman, "6 Reasons to Drink Water," WebMD, May 8, 2019, https://www.webmd.com/diet/features/6-reasons-to-drink-water#1.

CHAPTER 2: GET MOVING

1. James A. Blumenthal, Patrick J. Smith, and Benson M. Hoffman, "Is Exercise a Viable Treatment for Depression?," *ACSM's Health & Fitness Journal* 16,

no. 4 (July 2012): 14–21, https://www.ncbi.nlm.nih.gov/pmc/articles/PMC3674785/.

2. Therese Borchard, "Exercise Not Only Treats, but Prevents Depression," *The Second Pilgrimage* (blog), April 28, 2014, https://thereseborchard.com/exercise-not-only-treats-but-prevents-depression/.
3. Samuel B. Harvey et al., "Exercise and the Prevention of Depression: Results of the HUNT Cohort Study," *American Journal of Psychiatry* 175, no. 1 (January 2018): 28–36, https://ajp.psychiatryonline.org/doi/abs/10.1176/appi.ajp.2017.16111223?mobileUi=0&journalCode=ajp.
4. Alpa Patel, quoted at Janet Lee, "How Much Exercise Do You Need to Get Healthier?," *Consumer Reports*, updated February 20, 2019, https://www.consumerreports.org/exercise-fitness/how-much-exercise-do-you-need-to-see-health-benefits/.
5. U.S. Department of Health and Human Services, *Physical Activity Guidelines for Americans, 2nd edition* (Washington, DC: U.S. Department of Health and Human Services, 2018), https://health.gov/paguidelines/second-edition/pdf/Physical_Activity_Guidelines_2nd_edition.pdf.
6. Michael Bracko, quoted at Dulce Zamora, "Fitness 101: The Absolute Beginner's Guide to Exercise," WebMD, February 12, 2008, https://www.webmd.com/fitness-exercise/features/fitness-beginners-guide#1.
7. "How Does Exercise Help Those with Chronic Insomnia?," National Sleep Foundation, accessed June 11, 2024, https://sleepfoundation.org/ask

-the-expert/how-does-exercise-help-those-chronic-insomnia.

8. "Heart Disease Facts," Centers for Disease Control and Prevention, November 28, 2017, https://www.cdc.gov/heartdisease/facts.htm.
9. "Blood Glucose and Exercise," American Diabetes Association, September 25, 2017, http://www.diabetes.org/food-and-fitness/fitness/get-started-safely/blood-glucose-control-and-exercise.html.
10. Marily Oppezzo and Daniel L. Schwartz, "Give Your Ideas Some Legs: The Positive Effect of Walking on Creative Thinking," *Journal of Experimental Psychology: Learning, Memory, and Cognition* 40, no. 4 (July 2014): 1142–52, http://psycnet.apa.org/record/2014-14435-001.

CHAPTER 3: DEVELOP A SLEEP ROUTINE

1. "1 in 3 Adults Don't Get Enough Sleep," CDC Newsroom, CDC, last modified February 16, 2016, https://www.cdc.gov/media/releases/2016/p0215-enough-sleep.html. See also "Data and Statistics: Short Sleep Duration among US Adults," Sleep and Sleep Disorders, CDC, last modified May 2, 2017, https://www.cdc.gov/sleep/data_statistics.html.
2. National Sleep Foundation, *2011 Sleep in America® Poll: Communications Technology in the Bedroom* (Washington, DC: The Foundation, March 7, 2011), https://sleepfoundation.org/sites/default/files/sleepinamericapoll/SIAP_2011_Summary_of_Findings.pdf.

3. National Sleep Foundation, *2011 Sleep in America® Poll.*
4. "Nearly 7 in 10 Americans Are on Prescription Drugs," *ScienceDaily*, June 19, 2013, https://www.sciencedaily.com/releases/2013/06/130619132352.htm.
5. Harvard Health Publishing, "Insomnia in Later Life," *Harvard Mental Health Letter*, December 2006, https://www.health.harvard.edu/newsletter_article/Insomnia_in_later_life.
6. David Nutt, Sue Wilson, and Louise Paterson, "Sleep Disorders as Core Symptoms of Depression," *Dialogues in Clinical Neuroscience* 10, no. 3 (September 2008): 329–36, https://www.ncbi.nlm.nih.gov/pmc/articles/PMC3181883/.

CHAPTER 4: REDUCE STRESS

1. George M. Slavich and Michael R. Irwin, "From Stress to Inflammation and Major Depressive Disorder: A Social Signal Transduction Theory of Depression," *Psychological Bulletin* 140, no. 3 (May 2014): 774–815, https://www.ncbi.nlm.nih.gov/pmc/articles/PMC4006295/.
2. Janice K. Kiecolt-Glaser, Heather M. Derry, and Christopher P. Fagundes, "Inflammation: Depression Fans the Flames and Feasts on the Heat," *American Journal of Psychiatry* 172, no. 11 (November 1, 2015): 1075–91, https://ajp.psychiatryonline.org/doi/10.1176/appi.ajp.2015.15020152.
3. Norman B. Anderson, quoted at R. A. Clay, "Stressed in America," *Monitor on Psychology* 42, no. 1 (January

2011): 60, https://www.apa.org/monitor/2011/01/stressed-america.aspx.

4. Sammi R. Chekroud et al., "Association between Physical Exercise and Mental Health in 1.2 Million Individuals in the USA between 2011 and 2015: A Cross-Sectional Study," *Lancet Psychiatry* 5, no. 9 (August 8, 2018): 739–46, https://www.thelancet.com/journals/lanpsy/article/PIIS2215-0366(18)30227-X/fulltext.

CHAPTER 5: LIMIT TECHNOLOGY USE

1. Liu yi Lin et al., "Association between Social Media Use and Depression among U.S. Young Adults," *Depression and Anxiety* 33, no. 4 (April 2016): 323–31, https://www.ncbi.nlm.nih.gov/pmc/articles/PMC4853817/.
2. Phoebe Weston, "Are Teenagers Replacing Drugs and Alcohol with Technology? Experts Describe Smartphones as 'Digital Heroin' for Millennials," *Daily Mail*, March 14, 2017, http://www.dailymail.co.uk/sciencetech/article-4313278/Are-teenagers-replacing-drugs-alcohol-TECHNOLOGY.html.
3. Maeve Duggan, "Online Harassment 2017," Pew Research Center, July 11, 2017, http://www.pewinternet.org/2017/07/11/online-harassment-2017/.

CHAPTER 6: RELEASE ANGER, FEAR, AND GUILT

1. "Chronic Stress Puts Your Health at Risk," Mayo Clinic, April 21, 2016, https://www.mayoclinic.org/healthy-lifestyle/stress-management/in-depth/stress/art-20046037.

2. See "Forgiveness: Your Health Depends on It," Johns Hopkins Medicine, accessed January 7, 2019, https://www.hopkinsmedicine.org/health/healthy_aging/healthy_connections/forgiveness-your-health-depends-on-it. See also Everett L. Worthington Jr., ed., *Handbook of Forgiveness* (New York: Routledge, 2005), 355.

CHAPTER 7: PRACTICE SOUL CARE

1. Corporation for National and Community Service, Office of Research and Policy Development, *The Health Benefits of Volunteering: A Review of Recent Research* (Washington, DC, 2007), https://www.nationalservice.gov/pdf/07_0506_hbr.pdf.
2. S. L. Brown et al., "Providing Social Support May Be More Beneficial than Receiving It: Results from a Prospective Study of Mortality," *Psychological Science* 14, no. 4 (July 1, 2003): 320–27, https://www.ncbi.nlm.nih.gov/pubmed/12807404.

About the Authors

Gregory L. Jantz, PhD, is a popular speaker and award-winning author of many books, including *Healing the Scars of Emotional Abuse*, *Healing the Scars of Childhood Abuse*, and *Overcoming Anxiety, Worry, and Fear*. He is the founder of The Center: A Place of Hope, which was voted among the top ten clinics in the nation for healing depression. For more information about Dr. Jantz and The Center, please visit www.drgregoryjantz.com and www.aplaceofhope.com.

Keith Wall, a twenty-five-year publishing veteran, is an award-winning author, magazine editor, radio scriptwriter, and online columnist. He currently writes full time in collaboration with several bestselling authors. Keith lives in a mountaintop cabin near Manitou Springs, Colorado.